IT'S YOUR LIFE – A HEALTHY DIET MADE EASY

Professor Norman Ratcliffe

A catalogue record for this book is available from the British Library

ISBN: 978-1-907962-56-1

Published by Cranmore Publications

www.cranmorepublications.co.uk

This book is dedicated to my parents whose undying faith in my academic capabilities allowed me to pursue a scientific career. My gratitude also goes to my sister, Teri King, whose success as an author and constant encouragement and advice were such sources of inspiration. Thanks too to my many friends for tolerating so many mealtime discussions on health and diet as well as the unsolicited advice given to them!

Finally, I wish to thank Dr. Duncan McLaren of Swansea Metropolitan University for his outstanding enthusiasm and imagination during creation of sections of this book as well as Doreen Montgomery of Rupert Crew Ltd for her patient and helpful comments of the manuscript.

"IT'S YOUR LIFE"

THE AUTHOR

- **Professor Norman Ratcliffe** is a founder member of a team that recently discovered a new antibiotic potentially capable of curing MRSA and *Clostridium difficile*. This work was presented to Prince Phillip at St. James's Palace, London and was the subject of major media attention in the UK on ITV News and in many leading newspapers, including the Wall Street Journal, around the World. He is a Fellow of the Royal Society of Medicine and has previously run a "Health Alert" blood-testing company. He has published over 200 books and research papers on immunology, cancer invasion, influenza, tropical diseases and MRSA. He played squash for Wales, ran the London Marathon at the age of 50 and works-out regularly in the gym.

- **Professor Ratcliffe** retired recently after 25 years as a University Research Professor. He decided to finally complete "It's Your Life" after 5 years work in order to help the many people who are confused about health and fitness issues and who have constantly been asking his advice.

"IT'S YOUR LIFE"

THE SERIES

Professor Norman Ratcliffe's comprehensive book on health is: *It's Your Life: End the confusion from inconsistent health advice:*

www.cranmorepublications.co.uk/6

This book will often be referred to as IYL. Alongside this comprehensive book there is a series of smaller *It's Your Life: End the confusion from inconsistent health advice* books; this book is the first in the series. The aim of the series is to give advice to people in specific areas; all of the areas covered in the series are also included in IYL. The series is as follows:

It's Your Life – A Healthy Diet Made Easy

www.cranmorepublications.co.uk/61

It's Your Life – Avoiding Harmful Chemicals in Your Food

www.cranmorepublications.co.uk/62

It's Your Life – Avoid the Cocktail Effect of Harmful Chemicals in Your Body

www.cranmorepublications.co.uk/63

It's Your Life – Vitamins and Supplements For All Ages

www.cranmorepublications.co.uk/64

It's Your Life – Exercise For All Ages

www.cranmorepublications.co.uk/65

The main advice arising from IYL has also been summarised in:

117 Health Tips: A quick guide for a healthy life

www.cranmorepublications.co.uk/7

Contents

INTRODUCTION

A SIMPLE HEALTH PLAN

MIDDLE–AGE SPREAD, just look around it's everywhere. Can we avoid the weight-gain, diseases, degeneration and general malaise that often seem to accompany the aging process? Have you noticed, in recent years, how more and more young people appear middle-aged? Why are some diseases such as cancer of the colon and diabetes of such prominence now? Can we avoid these changes and diseases? This book does not profess to tell you how to live to be a 100 years old but it does show you, **SIMPLY,** how to maintain health and fitness and a feeling of well-being into your later years.

**Figure 1.   Showing slim (left) and overweight (right)
females for comparison. The
tape measure never lies!**

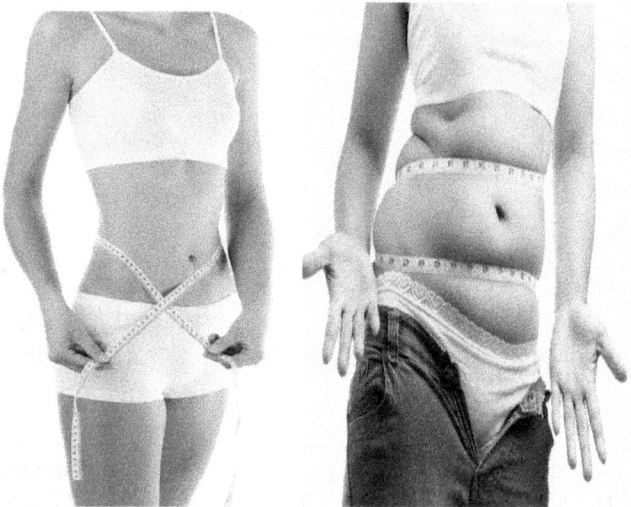

Figure 2.   Showing slim (left) and over weight (right), middle-aged men for comparison

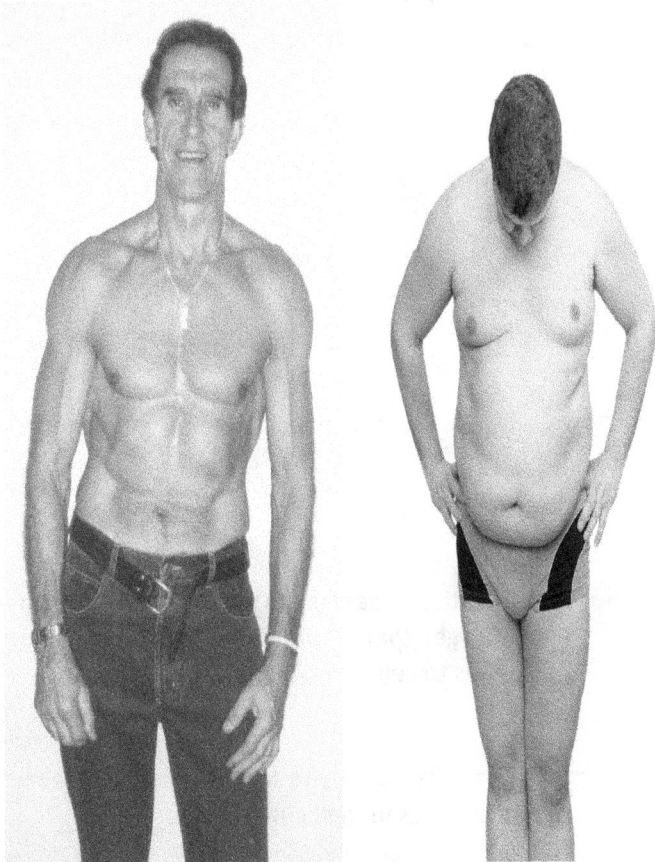

FED UP WITH THE CONSTANT BARRAGE OF HEALTH ADVICE AND DO'S AND DON'TS? The basics of a simple lifestyle are outlined on the next page. There is no need for you to read the entire book, you can simply try and follow the suggestions made in the 'Basic Health Plan'. If, however, you want to know more about the various components then the rest of the book will explain the details and will also introduce new health topics.

THE AGING PROCESS

Who knows why we age? Scientists have many theories including:

- Accumulation of damage to tissues by components of the oxygen that we breathe. Yes, oxygen can be poisonous to cells!

- Loss in ability of cells to multiply and self-repair due to changes in the aging chromosomes.

THE BASIC HEALTH PLAN

You have heard it all before from the media:

• Eat less junk-food and include 5 portions of fruit and vegetables in your diet each day
• Avoid too much animal fat and red meat - eat more fish and chicken
• Take regular exercise
• Give up smoking
• Avoid excess alcohol
• Examine your breasts, testicles and moles regularly for lumps and changes
• Get married

EASY TO SAY but how do you successfully change your lifestyle and end up with this desirable health plan? The following chapters will guide you **BUT REMEMBER :**

- If you hate reading health books then just concentrate on Chapter 1 ("Food, the basic diet") as this is designed as an introduction to a new health plan.

  Chapters 2 and 3 ("More about food" and "More facts about food, fat, fibre and fad diets") enlarge on Chapter 1 and tell you details about calories and important food components as well as changing your diet with age.

  Chapters 10 and 11 of IYL describe how to begin an exercise programme.

CHAPTER 1

FOOD

The Basic Diet (not dieting)

THERE IS NO NEED TO PILE ON THE POUNDS PAST 40 YEARS OLD

- It's getting more and more difficult to walk up those stairs, carry the shopping bags any distance, kick the ball around or make love. It's time to **take control**.

- You have abused your body with greasy breakfasts, hamburgers, chips, crisps, pasties, cakes, fizzy drinks and ready meals so that the pounds are piling on and you don't bother much with vegetables and fruit so **what can you do**?

- The fact that you are reading this book is a good start and shows that you are concerned. The best start you can make is simply to understand that **you are eating too many calories** and as you get older the extra calories will turn into ugly fatty deposits and block your heart and blood vessels. **REMEMBER, YOU ARE WHAT YOU EAT.**

First, what about breakfast? Those fry-ups are delicious aren't they? Can you slowly reduce the number that you have each week? Maybe down to just one on Saturday morning. If this is difficult then try having a few more beans or tomatoes instead of all that bacon, those two eggs, fried bread, chips and fat-filled mushrooms. **USE THE TOMATO KETCHUP** (do not worry about snooty waiters). Ketchup is particularly good for men.

There is evidence that the red pigment, lycopene, an antioxidant found in tomatoes, and to a lesser extent in apricots, pink grapefruits, papayas and guavas, can protect against cancer of the prostate in men. A number of so-called "epidemiological studies" which looked at dietary intake of lycopene from tomatoes and tomato products and incidence rates of prostate cancer, found a reduced risk of cancer. One such study involved nearly 48,000 men over 12 years and reported that 2+ servings of tomato or tomato products per week significantly reduced prostate cancers rates (see reference 1).

Needless to say, there are other scientific studies that disagree about the protective properties of lycopene. The US Food and Drug Administration reviewed all these studies and concluded that there is "limited evidence to support an association between tomato consumption and reduced risks of prostate, ovarian, gastric, and pancreatic cancers" (see reference 2).

TOMATO SAUCE HAS PARTICULARLY HIGH LEVELS OF LYCOPENE which is highly concentrated during heating of the tomatoes to release this red pigment from the tissues. The oil base of the sauce assists lycopene absorption in the gut. Other food products containing high levels of lycopene include tomato juice, tomato paste, condensed tomato soup, pizza sauce, spaghetti and baked bean sauce and some barbecue sauces. Raw tomatoes are best cooked to release the lycopene.

Figure 1. Who says that a dog is man's best friend? Tomatoes contain high levels of the red pigment, lyco-pene, which can significantly reduce rates of prostate cancer in men

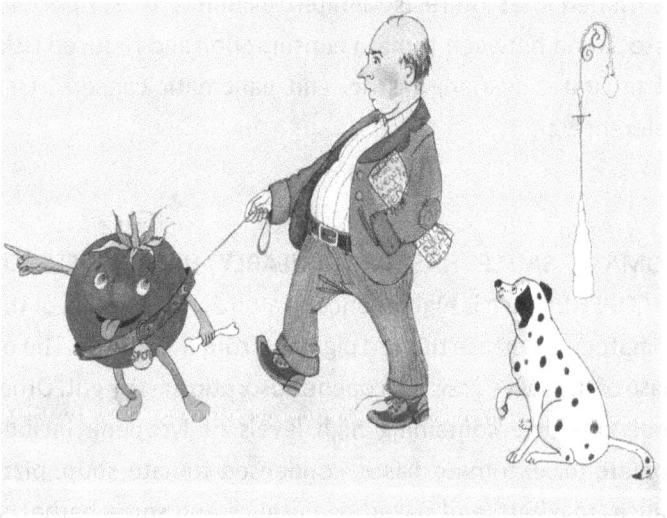

NEVER MISS BREAKFAST COMPLETELY as it is, as the name implies, the breaking of the overnight fasting and your blood sugar levels will be low. Your sugar levels will continue to fall and, unless you eat something, you will be tempted to snack mid-morning. What can you eat **instead of fried breakfasts or white toast with thick layers of butter or margarine or no breakfast at all?** Some cereal (Weetabix, Shredded Wheat or unsweetened Muesli are much better than Sugar Puffs, Cornflakes, Rice Crispies or Coco Pops) with skimmed milk is good, maybe with a little toast (wholemeal is best) and marmalade/Marmite. Try the toast just with marmalade/jam/Marmite and you will soon forget about the butter/margarine. Significantly, Marks and Spencer are removing products made with **trans fats (=hydrogenated vegetable fats, causing heart problems, see Chapter 3 for details), including some MARGARINES, from the shelves.** Try and avoid whole milk in latte or cappuccino. When ordering a coffee in a restaurant, it is worthwhile asking what sort of milk is being used and requesting skimmed or semi-skimmed if possible.

If you are really determined to start anew then **OATMEAL PORRIDGE (** which has low fat and salt, and reduces cholesterol and stress) with skimmed milk and a little honey is great, not only for the heart but also will suppress the desire to snack later in the day.

The importance of breakfast for children cannot be overemphasised.

A recent survey of 213 children between the ages of 4 and 11 commissioned by Kellogg's entitled "The Effects of Cereal on Children" (detailed at **www.kelloggs.co.uk/mediacentre**) showed that children who eat cereal for breakfast are mentally more alert for school than children who skip breakfast. The benefits of eating breakfast cereal included:

Benefits of children eating breakfast cereal before school

- 9 percent more alert
- 11 percent less emotionally distressed
- 13 percent less tired
- 17 percent less anxious
- 10 percent less likely to suffer memory and attention span problems
- 33 percent less likely to suffer from stomach complaints

Eating breakfast results in higher concentration and energy levels, as well as improving behaviour and well-being in children.

Figure 2. Shows that eating breakfast results in higher concentration and better school work in children as well as increased energy levels and improved behaviour and well-being.

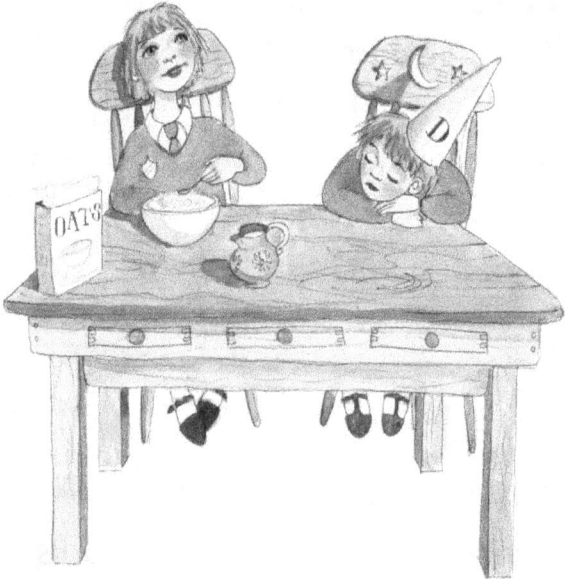

No, don't go on a **NEW FAD OR TRENDY DIET** that you read about in the newspaper or your favorite celebrity is promoting for money. First, just try replacing the fizzy drink with water or non-fizzy fruit juice (but not too many as juices contain calories too) and introduce an apple, orange, banana or a few grapes (any fruit!) into your diet each day. Once you succeed then look at the hamburger, cheeseburger, chips, meat pie, instant frozen meal or white roll etc that you normally eat and **consult the calorie chart (see Chapter 2, Table 1).** Do you really want all that processed high fat and salt-containing stodge or could you replace it with a few potatoes or rice (brown preferred) and a piece of cooked chicken or fish? Sounds boring but can be delicious with some pasta sauce on the chicken/fish cooked (not burnt) in a pan/oven with olive oil.

AVOID EATING RED MEAT EVERY DAY as it has been estimated that people who eat red meat twice instead of once per week have double the chance of developing bowel cancer. Recently, it has been shown that men who ate high amounts of red meat per week (about 6 oz or more =160 grams red meat per day) were 22% more likely to die from cancer and 27% more likely to die from heart disease than those who ate low amounts of red meat (about 1 oz = 25 grams) per day. In women, the equivalent figures for those who eat high amounts of red meat were 20% more likely to die of <u>cancer</u> and 50% more likely to die of heart disease, compared with women who consumed the lowest levels. Processed meats such as hotdogs, sausages and pepperoni were even worse than red meat (see reference 3).

By all means have a good steak or roast beef once a week. Red meat includes beef, lamb, bacon, gammon and pork, while white meats are chicken, turkey and fish. White meat should be eaten most days although the occasional omelette is fine.

FANTASTIC, YOU ARE WELL ON THE WAY.

Next try and include a few peas, beans, carrots (fresh cooked are delicious) or any vegetable you can stand with your meal. Yes, cooking is a chore so salad is fine or **buy a steamer** in which you can cook all the vegetables individually in the separate pans (retaining their vitamins) all at one time with minimal washing up (See Chapter 7 of IYL, pages 148-9, for hints on the best methods of cooking to retain vitamins).

Again, but **especially men**, always use the ketchup freely (see pages 20-22 for reasons).

Whatever you do, try and watch the **amount of salt** that you are eating (see reference 4).

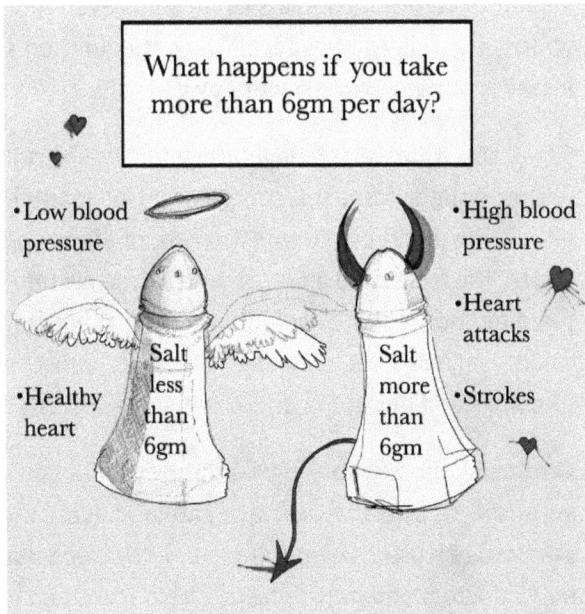

Figure 3. Shows that excess salt raises blood pressure and causes strokes and heart disease

The recommended daily amount is about 6 grams which is just more than one level teaspoon. Most salt is eaten in processed meals, crisps, bread, sauces and soup (see Chapter 2, Table 1, for salt contents of many foods). Read the labels on foods and remember the **"sodium" levels** shown have to be **multiplied by 2.5** in order to arrive at the true salt content. You will soon realize that a single instant meal often contains as much or even more than your 6 gram daily allowance! Thus, the limit on sodium intake is about 2.5 grams per day.

What about desserts? Have you tried **fresh fruit salad** (either bought from the supermarket or made by you) with some low fat yoghurt? You cannot stand yoghurt!? Ok, try the fruit salad alone or with a little custard or rice pudding (not made with full fat milk!). There is no fruit salad available? Ok, skip the rolly polly and chocolate puddings and buy some dried fruit and nuts instead.

Gradually, modify your diet, as above, until you will be surprised to find that you are eating at least the "**five portions of fruit or vegetables every day**" recommended by all doctors and nutritionists. These fruits and vegetables will contain most of the vitamins and minerals needed and all of the fibre required for a healthy gut (see Chapter 3 for more details on fibre).

**Figure 4. Shows the benefits of eating at least 5 portions
of fruit and vegetables per day**

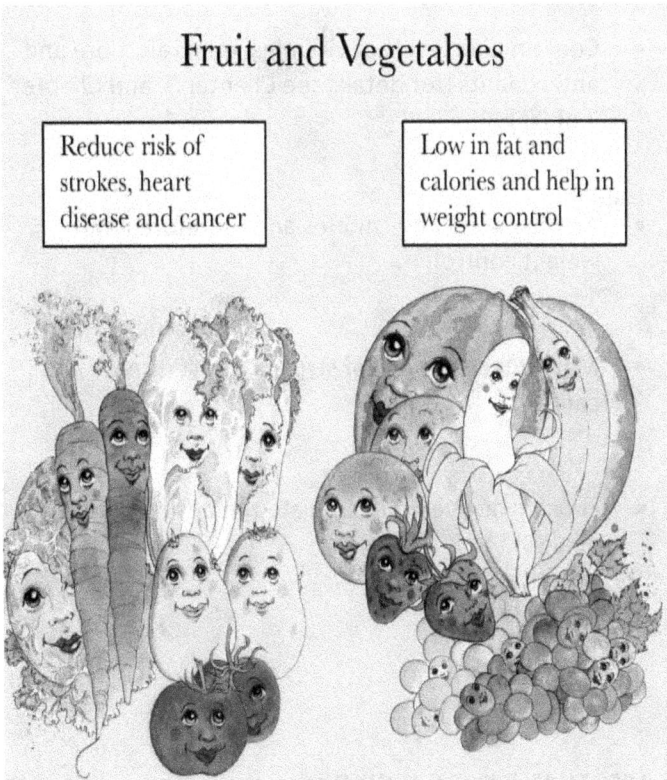

Fruit and Vegetables

Reduce risk of strokes, heart disease and cancer

Low in fat and calories and help in weight control

We are constantly told to eat 5 portions of fruit or vegetables per day for a number of reasons since they:

- Contain high levels of vitamins, minerals, fibre and antioxidants (for details see Chapter 3, and Chapter 7 of IYL)

- Are low in fat and calories and therefore help weight control

- May reduce the risk of strokes, heart disease and cancer

- Look attractive and stimulate the desire to eat healthily

LESS THAN 50% OF PEOPLE are aware of the need to eat 5 portions of fruit and vegetables every day. This is despite the constant reminder to do so by the media and health advisors.

EVEN FEWER PEOPLE know what makes up a portion of fruit or vegetable

SO WHAT IS A PORTION? It is no good being told to eat "5 portions" unless we know exactly what makes up a portion. According to the Food Standards Agency (**www.eatwell.gov.uk/healthydiet** and **www.5aday.nhs.uk/whatcounts**) :

A PORTION OF FRUIT OR VEGETABLES = 80 g or just less than 3 ounces

However, we cannot weigh (especially in restaurants) all the fruit and vegetables that we eat so try remembering that **a portion** (fresh, tinned or frozen) is:

- 1 small glass (150ml or about 1/3 pint) of fruit or vegetable juice or smoothie* but fruit juice only counts as one portion no matter how many glasses you drink

- 2 smaller fruits such as plums, tangerines, kiwi fruits, or 3 apricots

- 1 medium fruit such as apple, pear, orange, nectarine or banana

- for larger fruits – ½ a grapefruit or avocado or 1 slice of melon or pineapple or 2 slices of mango (all about 2-inches thick)

- a handful of grapes, berries or dried fruit

- 3 heaped tablespoons of vegetables, chopped fruit or pulses (beans, peas, and lentils). Again, pulses only count as one portion no matter how much you eat.

- A small dessert bowl of salad

* Smoothies are very fashionable and can be beneficial but **take care to check their   ingredients** since they can have high sugar, fat and calorie contents. Also, most of the fibre has been removed and sometimes they are mixed with whole fat milk or yoghurt and not made with fresh fruit but fruit concentrate containing fewer vitamins and minerals. The famous American Peanut Butter Moo'd, marketed by Jumba Juice, contains chocolate and peanut butter and every 890ml packet has 1170 calories and 169 grams of sugars!

Potatoes are starchy foods and do not count towards your 5 portions per day.

If possible, drink a glass of red wine with dinner as it is good for the heart and circulation too.

DRINK PLENTY OF WATER throughout the day as it will help to detoxify the body, prevent dehydration, constipation and fatigue. Who counts how much they drink? However, about 6-8 average glasses of fluid per day is recommended and water, milk, teas, coffee, soup and fruit juices all count. Normal teas and coffees do tend to dehydrate the body and if your urine becomes dark yellow then drink some more water. The above 6-8 glasses of fluid per day apply whether you eat at home or in the canteen in work but do not count any alcohol.

THE TAP WATER VERSUS BOTTLED WATER DEBATE

See pages 52-57 of this chapter

Yes, the above looks like a diet but it is just sensible eating. The important thing is **NOT TO CHANGE EVERYTHING AT ONCE** but just pick those things that are easiest for you and introduce them slowly so that they become part of your normal daily routine. Following the advice above you should end up with a so-called **"Balanced Diet"**.

A balanced diet would include the following food groups:

1. **Bread, cereals, pasta, rice and potatoes** which are high in carbohydrate and called "starchy" foods. Carbohydrate should make up 50-60% of calories in diet.

2. **Fruit and vegetables** since these contain healthy carbohydrate, protein (pulses), fibre and vitamins.

3. **Meat** as a source of protein to include red meat, poultry, fish, eggs, and meat substitutes such as nuts and pulses (peas, beans and lentils). Avoid too much red meat (beef, pork, ham, lamb) and eat no more than 1-2 times per week. Protein to make up 15-25 % of calories in diet.

4. **Milk and dairy products** to include milk, cheese and yoghurt (all low-fat or skimmed) provide some protein, calcium and B vitamins and fats. Fats to make up 10-15% of calories in diet.

5. **Soft drinks and foods** such as sweets, jam, cakes, biscuits, puddings, crisps, ice cream and sauces all contain high added sugar and/or saturated fats and **should be limited and reduced if possible.**

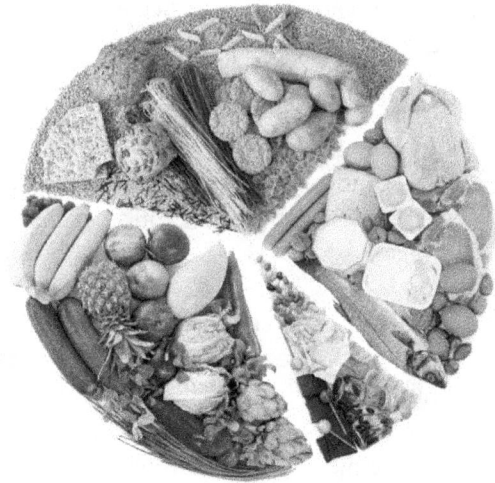

Figure 5. Shows the main groups of foods described above. The size of each slice represents the proportion of the diet that should contain that food group. Hence the smallest slice contains sweets, biscuits, cakes etc. Note that meat and dairy products have been combined into one slice

- A "balanced diet" would include a combination of foods from all of the main food groups (above) at each meal.

- Avoid foods high in saturated fat and trans fats as well as those with high levels of added sugar and salt (see Chapters 2 and 3).

- Beware added salt with a limit of 6 grams per day (= about one teaspoon full) or no more than 2.5 grams of sodium. This is confusing since sodium and not salt is often shown on food labels instead of salt (why do supermarkets do this?).

- There is no need to go on a special diet. Just gradually introduce healthy options into your diet to replace high fat, salt and sugar containing foods.

Figure 6. Shows junk food on the right-hand scale gradually being replaced by healthy fruit and vegetables on the left-hand scale to eventually arrive at a balanced diet

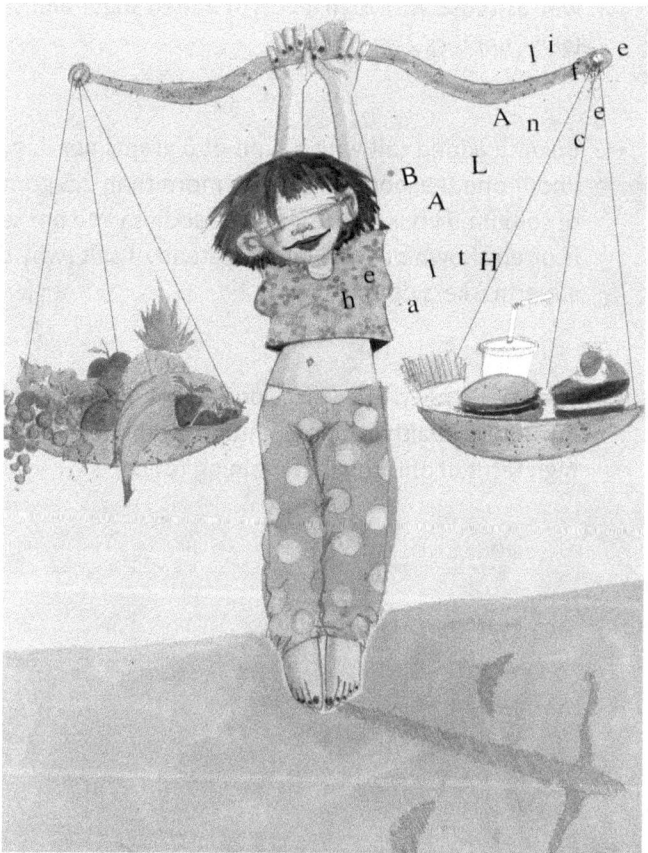

Do not beat yourself up mentally if you lapse with your diet as your new exercise regime (see Chapters 9-11 of IYL) will more than compensate for the odd uncontrollable urge. Also, it has been shown that junk food rich in fat and sugar can be **addictive** just like tobacco or other drugs so **MAKE GRADUAL CHANGES**.

- **I CAN HEAR SOME OF YOU SAYING:**

- "but my diet is healthy and I am still overweight"

or

- " I saw that television program on people inheriting a "fat gene"* and I think that
I am one of those people"

or even

41

- "I have a slow metabolic rate, I just look at food and the pounds go on".

GENERALLY, NONE OF THESE ARE WHOLLY TRUE AND WHAT IS HAPPENING IS THAT YOUR DAILY ACTIVITY IS NOT USING UP ENOUGH OF THE CALORIES TAKEN IN WITH YOUR FOOD.

This imbalance can change rapidly at different times in your life such as following **marriage**, during **pregnancy**, as you **age** and stop participating in sport, or even as the **children grow up** or following the **death of the dog**. Similar inertia can result from **depression** and the **breakup of a marriage**, **retirement**, **illness**, **bereavement** and a **change of job**.

This decreased physical activity, for whatever reason, will result in a loss in muscle mass. Then, since the muscles are the most metabolically active (i.e. calorie-burning) tissue in the body, their loss will result in increased weight unless your food/calorie intake is reduced.

*See, for example, reference 5 for details of the so-called "fat gene".

Figure 7. Shows some of the reasons for declines in physical activity

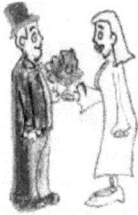

Marriage

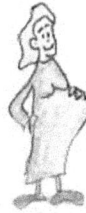

Pregnancy

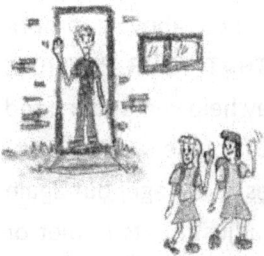

Children grown up

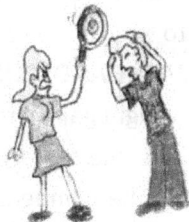

Divorce

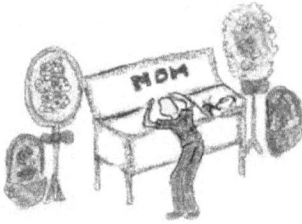

Bereavement

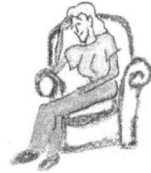

Depression

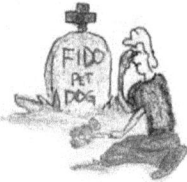

Death of dog

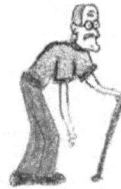

Aging

Why not sit down and tick off any of the above appropriate to you or other **REASONS THAT YOUR PHYSICAL ACTIVITY HAS DECLINED?** This may help you understand your weight gain in recent years. Of course, we lose muscle mass due to hormonal changes as we age, but again this can be compensated for by adjustments in diet or exercise regimes (see Chapter 2 and Chapters 9-11 of IYL).

Finally, since we are trying to **BE REALISTIC** here, I can hear you saying that the simple healthy food options described above "will take **too much time to prepare**". It's much easier to run down to MacDonalds or the chip shop and stoke up with junk food before getting on with the more important things in life. There is no easy answer to this except to say that **FEW THINGS ARE MORE IMPORTANT IN LIFE THAN GOOD HEALTH**. Ignore this fact at your peril as father time catches up with us all but **much sooner than later** if you neglect your body.

If you simply cannot change your diet, then try eating the same things but in smaller portions. This will result in considerable weight loss and encourage you to modify your diet and eat healthier. Remember, you may not be particularly overweight but still be eating junk and have elevated levels of unhealthy fats such as dangerous types of cholesterol. These in turn will block your arteries and increase your risk of heart disease.

DAILY CALORIE REQUIREMENTS OF MEN AND WOMEN*.
To generalize, the number of calories needed by women to maintain body weight is **2000 kcal** while for men it is higher at **2500 kcal**. These are very broad generalizations and will vary significantly according to your sex, age, height, weight and daily activity levels. People with lean muscular bodies who exercise regularly will need more calories than fatter people who are less active. Men also tend to need more calories than women. There are numerous tables for calculating your daily calorie requirements and your result will vary according to the table used (for example, see:

www.realage.com/NutritionCenter/calorieCount.aspx

which is very useful since the calculation includes not only your height, weight, sex and level of activity but also your age). A quick calculation sometimes given is to:

For men: multiply your weight in lbs by 14

For women: multiply your weight in lbs by 12

Examples:

187 lbs (85 kilo) elderly male   =   187 x 14 = 2618 kcal

132 lbs (60 kilo) elderly female =   132 x 12 = 1584 kcal

These results are extremely general since the calorie requirements shown are very low and only accurate for elderly people who are not very active. Increase the activity and decrease the age and much higher calorie requirements will be obtained (see also Chapter 2, page 66).

A recent report by the Scientific Advisory Committee on Nutrition (SACN), a committee of independent experts that advises the Food Standards Agency and Department of Health, has found that present calculations of calorie requirements are underestimated by approximately 16% (see reference 6). Thus, the 2000 kcal recommended for women would be 2320 kcal.

This **does not mean** that we can all go and eat an extra cheeseburger per day. This revised calculation resulted from an underestimate of the average physical activity of people in the UK, particularly for routine activities of daily living on energy expenditure. The report is only in draft form, will cause confusion and has yet to be approved.

ALWAYS REMEMBER WEIGHT GAIN OCCURS WHEN

"CALORIES EATEN EXCEED CALORIES USED BY BODY"

**For example, every day eat 500 less kcal +
take more exercise = weight loss**

TO LOSE WEIGHT all you will have to do is reduce food intake by 500 kcal per day (3500 per week) or exercise more. Why not combine the two and cut out a mince pie, a packet of crisps or reduce food portion size (each about 250 calories less) and cycle or walk briskly for 30 min per day or for a longer time 2-3 times per week. Any combination will reduce/burn more calories.

- **BEWARE - Do not reduce food intake too quickly at the same time as you are increasing exercise or you will greatly stimulate your appetite.**

BODY MASS INDEX (BMI)

Body Mass Index is a useful way of determining if you are overweight and calculating the ideal weight for your height. BMI can be calculated as follows:

BMI = your weight in kilograms divided by your height in metres squared

- **Example 1:** woman weighing 60 kg (132 lb = 9 stone 4.3 lb) and 1.7 m (5ft 7in) tall

$$BMI = \frac{60}{1.7 \times 1.7} = \frac{60}{2.89} = 20.76$$

- **Example 2:** man weighing 85 kilos (187 lb = 13 stone 3.4 lb) and 1.88 m (6ft 2in) tall

$$BMI = \frac{85}{1.88 \times 1.88} = \frac{85}{3.53} = 24$$

BMI Categories

- less than 18.5	=	underweight
- 18.5 to 25	=	normal weight
- 25 to 30	=	overweight
- 30 to 40	=	obese
- over 40	=	very obese

NB: Sometimes BMI can be misleading so that men with well developed muscles, such as rugby players or athletes , may have high BMIs and be classified as overweight or even obese which, of course, they are not.

TAP WATER OR BOTTLED WATER?

According to the **Drinking Water Inspectorate** (DWI, http://www.dwi.gov.uk) in 2003, 2.9 million tests of tap water were undertaken and 99.88 % passed. **This does mean that 3,480 failed**. Also, outbreaks of the diarrhoea parasite, *Cryptosporidium,* in 2006 are still fresh in the minds of many people in Wales. In 1988, the population of the Cornish town of Camelford also drank water contaminated with excessively high levels of aluminium sulphate accidentally added to the tap water. Subsequently, on the basis of the post-mortem of just one person dying, the suggestion has been made that this incident was linked to the development of an Alzheimer's-like disease in this patient. The DWI also monitors tap water for **bacteria, pesticides, nitrates from fertilizers, and metals such as lead.** All of these substances have been reported, in a small number of tap water samples, to exceed safety levels (see details in "Water Quality in Your Region" at www.dwi.gov.uk).

- **SHOULD WE THEREFORE ONLY DRINK BOTTLED WATER?**

- **IT IS NOT THAT SIMPLE SINCE:**

- **There are different forms of bottled water:**

i. Mineral Water which is natural, untreated and from a named source identified on the label. The addition of minerals is not allowed. Babies and young children should not drink mineral water due to high salt or sulphur content.

ii. Spring Water is again from a named source shown on the label but it may have minerals added or be artificially carbonated.

iii. Bottled Water in which the source is not identified and could be from the tap as with PepsiCo's Aquafina . Many bottled waters are just **filtered tap water** with the chlorine removed. **Crystal Spring**, for example, was produced from tap water in the basement of a London restaurant! **Flavoured Waters** should be avoided due to their content of artificial sweeteners, including aspartame and acesulphame, as well as preservatives like benzoic acid (see Chapter 5 of IYL "Additives, Preservatives and Colourants", for more details).

UNFORTUNATELY, it has been shown that bottled water of all types can be contaminated with bacteria, fungi, synthetic organic chemicals, arsenic etc (see: http://www.nrdc.org/water/drinking/nbw.asp for details) The latest example was in July 2007, when the Foods Standard Agency (http://www.food.gov.uk/news/pressreleases/2007/jul/bottledwater) alerted consumers to the risk of bacterial contamination in Hadham Naturally Pure English Spring Water which was then removed from sale.

IN ADDITION, there are reports that toxic chemicals can be absorbed from the plastic containers into the bottled water. One such toxic substance is antimony which was shown to leach very rapidly from the plastic into the water when stored for just 3 months. **The sell by dates of many bottled waters, of all 3 types, is often 1-2 years!** Antimony could potentially be very dangerous as are other chemicals that can leach out of the plastic container. These include phalates which are released from the plastic if the bottle is filled with acidic fruit juice and are cancer forming and hormone disruptors (see Chapter 6 of IYL "The Cocktail Effect").

CONCLUSIONS, from the above, it is obvious why people are confused. The author's opinion is that it is simply not worthwhile buying bottled water of any description because:

1. There is little evidence that bottled is purer than tap water in the UK

2. Due to 1-2 year storage before drinking, dangerous chemicals could potentially leach into the water from the plastic and the environment

3. It costs too much

4. The plastic bottles are either thrown everywhere or incinerated to liberate dioxins and are an environmental disaster

5. It is simply insane to generate high levels of carbon in the manufacturing of plastic bottles and their transportation from country to country

6. Due to high levels of minerals in some bottled water, it should not be given to babies and young children and should not be used to make up baby feeds

7. Do not be afraid to ask for tap water in restaurants but remember they are entitled (would you believe) to charge you for the ice and service.

THE BEST COMPROMISE IS PROBABLY TO BUY A WATER FILTRATION SYSTEM with the cheapest with a filter (Brita, Wilkinson etc) that slots into a plastic (!) reservoir. Water can be rapidly filtered and then decanted into a glass bottle and stored in the refrigerator. The filter should be changed regularly (every month) to avoid growth of bacteria trapped by the filter. Such simple filters will significantly reduce metal contaminants including lead from plumbing and aluminium from water treatment plants but are less effective against copper or fluoride. They also remove chlorine but **not** some of the harmful by-products of chlorine but these evaporate off the filtered water after storage for several hours. The best option is to install a proper water filtration system above the sink. This, however, can be expensive, but if you are concerned about possible toxic effects of fluoride added to the tap water then a portable reverse osmosis filter can be bought for about £150 and is easily fitted (www.eastmidlandswater.co.uk). There is a very active ongoing debate about the advantages/disadvantages of water fluoridation but even bottled water may have significant levels of fluoride. Water fluoridation is now banned in the majority of countries in Europe but still carried out in areas of the UK (see: http://www.dwi.gov.uk/consumer/fluoridemaps.pdf for details in your area). The author has no connection with any water filtration company.

SUMMARY FOR A HEALTHIER DIET AND WEIGHT CONTROL

• BE DETERMINED TO CHANGE
• AVOID FAD DIETS
• EAT BREAKFAST
• STOP SNACKING
• SELECT HEALTHY FOODS WITH LOWER FAT AND SALT
• GET RID OF PROCESSED FOOD FROM THE DIET
• GET ENOUGH FIBRE
• EAT AT LEAST 5 PORTIONS OF VEGETABLES OR FRUIT EACH DAY
• DRINK PLENTY OF WATER
• MAKE CHANGES GRADUALLY
• LIST REASONS FOR DECLINE IN PHYSICAL ACTIVITY

REMEMBER to change your life-style slowly so that your new diet and exercise regimens become a natural part of everyday living.

CHAPTER 2

MORE ABOUT FOOD

HELP! WHAT AM I EATING?

Table 1 (see page 68) lists the **calorie, fat, salt and sugar** content of different types of food and will help in planning a healthier diet. It will assist in identifying those foods and snacks that are a **danger to your health** and really should be eliminated or reduced in the diet. Table 1 **also gives the fibre content** of foods as a further assistance in selecting a healthy diet (see Chapter 3 for "Facts About Fibre").

HOW TO USE TABLE 1

The colour coding in Table 1 is based upon the Food Standards Agency's **TRAFFIC LIGHT COLOURS** (see reference 7).

In Table 1 these colours are converted into different shades of grey/white, as below:

DARK GREY	High Levels**
MEDIUM GREY	Medium Levels
LIGHT GREY/WHITE	Low Levels	Very Low Levels[+]

** The stars in the dark grey colour draw attention to **very high levels** of calories, fat, salt and sugar. The more stars the higher the levels.

+ The light grey/white colour is used to draw attention to those foods that are **very low in harmful substances** such as saturated fats or **very high in beneficial fibre**.

The dark grey colour indicates those foods that have an excess of harmful calories, fat, salt or sugar and which should be reduced in your diet

The medium grey colour indicates those foods that do not contain an excess of harmful calories, fat, salt or sugar but should occasionally be replaced by healthier options

The light grey/white colour indicates those foods that are low or very low in harmful nutrients or high in beneficial fibre. The more of these foods you have the healthier your diet.

A SIMPLE EXAMPLE OF HOW TO USE TABLE 1

(see page 68 for Table 1)

- Patients who have suffered heart attacks or strokes often have **high blood pressure** (hypertension) and are advised to reduce their daily intake of salt as well as to adopt a low-fat diet.

- It has, however, been calculated that **processed foods** (rather than the salt pot) may account for **75% of the daily consumption of salt**.

- It is therefore vitally important to be able to **identify those foods with high salt levels** and to eliminate them from the diet.

- Using Table 1, it is easy and very rapid to identify the high salt-containing foods just by **looking down the column labelled "Salt Grams"**.

- All foods with **high salt contents will be identified in dark grey**. For some foods, the results are not surprising as with high salt in ready meals and burgers but **salt is also present but hidden in other foods,** such as some breads, sandwiches and breakfast cereals.

- **Do take into account the amount of a particular food eaten** i.e. the number of slices of bread or ounces or grams when estimating your salt intake. The weights of each food from which levels of calories, fat etc have been calculated are given in the far left column, alongside the name of the food.

- Table 1 does not include the over 50,000 different foods found in supermarkets but includes the main groups of food so that reasonable estimates can be made. (for additional foods not in Table 1, see references 8-10).

- The same simple exercise of looking down the appropriate column and reading off the name of the food can be done for checking on calories, fat, saturated fat, fibre and sugar.

CASE STUDY -THE AUTHOR

Even the author does not completely eliminate dark grey coloured foods shown in Table 1 and he has a particular weakness for dark chocolate and chocolate biscuits. After all, **life has to be worth living,** especially when writing a book over a number of years. It is a question of controlling these urges, being aware of which foods contain harmful levels of fats, salt and sugar and only eating these **occasionally**.

The following is a guideline to the number of calories* required daily and limits on the daily consumption of fat, saturated fat, salt and sugar.

"Average" Woman**	"Average" Man**
(ca. 63.5 kilo (140 lbs), 25 yr old, 5ft 4" tall, active)	(ca. 73 kilo (161 lbs), 25 yr old, 5ft 8" tall, active)
Calories 2300 kcal*** Fat 70 g Saturated fat 20 g Salt 6 g Added sugar 50 g	Calories 3000 kcal*** Fat 95 g Saturated fat 30 g Salt 6 g Added sugar 70 g

* Each kilocalorie (kcal) = 1000 calories, and the term "kilocalorie" and "Calorie" (with large "C" often written as "Cal") are the same thing". Some articles on nutrition sometimes use calorie (small "c") to mean kcal which is confusing. In Table 1 "Calories" refers to "kcal".

** The number of calories, fats and sugar required will, of course, vary according to how much the person weighs, as well as their age and the amount of exercise taken daily (see also Chapter 1, page 46).

*** Note, the recent recalculations of calorie require-ments discussed in Chapter 1, page 47.

Table 1. SHOWING CALORIE, FAT, SALT, FIBRE AND SUGAR CONTENTS OF SOME COMMON FOODS.

Type of Food[1]	Calories	Fat grams (of which satu-rates)	Salt grams	Fibre grams	Sugar grams
FISH ▶	Most fish are low in harmful saturated fats, salt and sugar but note high saturated fats in battered fish and scampi ▼				
Cod fillet , 100g (3.5oz)	80	0.7 (0.1)[2]	0.3	0	0
Cod, Young's, battered, frozen, 1 fillet, ca.137g	271	15.6 (8)		1.7	0.5
Herring, (=kipper), Scottish hot smoked fillet, 1 typical, 80g	205	15.8 (3.8)	1.6	0	0
Lemon sole, 1 fillet 150g	125	2.3 (0.3)	0.5	0	0

Lemon sole, breaded, 1 fillet, 160g	330	14.2 (1.4)	1.7	2.2	2.9
Scottish Mackerel Tesco, 1 fillet, 100g	310	24.9 (6.7)	1.9	0	0
Mussels, ½ live pot, 140g	141	5.6 (3.5)	0.7	1.4	1.8
Prawns, Tesco, cooked and peeled, 100g	72	0.6 (0.1)	1.5	0	0
Rainbow trout, 1 x 140g	231	14.3 (3.4)	0.4	0.7	0
Salmon farmed, 1 fillet, 130g	265	17.7 (4)	0.25	0	0
Sardines, Princes, in tomato sauce, 100g	190	11.9 (3.3)	1.25	0	1.6
Sardines, Princes, in olive oil, 100g	222	13.9 (3.1)	1.25	0	0
Scampi, Young's, frozen, 100g	219	12.4 (6.5)	1.2	2.1	1.9
Seafood collection, Tesco, mussels, crab, prawns, 100g	105	2.2 (0.7)	1.05	0	0.7

Tuna chunks, sunflower oil, drained, one small can, 185g, (6.5oz)	270	12.6 (2)	0.5	0	0
MEAT/MEAT PRODUCTS	Note very high calorie, saturated fat levels and salt in some mince, pies, sausages and McDonalds ▼ ▼			
Beef rump steak (fat trimmed) 200g (7oz)	307	7.2 (3)	0.3	0	0.2
Chicken mini breasts, skinned, 200g (7oz)	206	2 (0.6)	0.6	0	0
Chicken thighs – one 165g (6oz)	174	7.8 (2)	0.2	0	0
Duck, 125g (4.4oz) roasted	334	27.8 (7.8)	0.3	0	0
Lamb, Welsh, 2 chops (fat trimmed), 84g	150	6.4 (3.4)	0.3	0	0.1
Lamb, Welsh, leg, roasted (fat trimmed), 100g	175	8.2 (4.2)	0.4	0	0.1

Pork rump steak (fat trimmed) 200g (7oz)	273	7.4 (3)	0.3	0	0
Turkey, breast, fillet medallions, 100g	110	1.2 (0.6)	0.3	0	0
Mince, pork, 225g (8oz)	288	10.4 (4)	0.3	0	0
Mince, steak, lean 225g (8oz)	418	13.3 (6)	0.45	0	0.1
Mince, beef, 225g (8oz)	720	63 (29) ***	0.35	0	0.1
Mince, lamb, 225g (8oz)	518	40 (20) ***	0.35	0	0.1
Bacon, thick cut back, 2 grilled rashers, 54g	175	14.1 (4.7)	2.3	0	0
Faggots, pork, Mr. Brains, frozen, 2 ca. 188g	256	12.2 (4.8)	2.8	1.6	1.2
Pate, Tesco smooth, Brussels, 50g	164	15.9 (6.1)	1	0.8	0.4

Pate, Tesco Healthy Living, Brussels, 50g	100	7.6 (3.2)	1	1	0
Pie, pork, Melton Mowbray, small, 140g (5oz)	535	35 (13)*	1.6	0	4.2
Pie, steak and ale, deep fill, puff pastry, per 150g (5.4 oz)	344	20 (8.7)	1	2.8	1.3
Pie, steak pie, 150g (5.4 oz)	445	27 (13)*	1.5	3.8	1.7
Sausages, pork and Bramley apple, 2 grilled	386	29 (12)*	1.8	1.8	9.5
Sausages, thick pork , 2 grilled	225	13 (4.7)	2	1.7	1.1
Sausages, finest chunky Cumberland pork, 1 grilled	266	20 (7.7)	1.3	1	2.1
Sausages, beef, 2 grilled	270	18 (7.3)	1.8	0	0.5
Scotch eggs, snack, two =90g (3oz)	270	18 (5)	1.4	1.6	0
McDonalds Hamburger, 100g (3.5oz)	250	8 (3)	1.2	3	7

McDonalds Big Mac, 214g (7.5oz)	495	23 (10)*	2	5.3	8.9
McDonalds Cheeseburger, 100g (3.5oz)	300	12 (6)	1.5	3	8
McDonalds Quarter Pounder with cheese, 100g, (3.5 oz)	515	25 (12)*	1.2	4	9
McDonalds Big Tasty	840***	50 (21)***			
McDonalds Big Mac + Large Fries + Large Milk Shake!!!!!!!!	1470***	59 (21)***	3.5	12.3	92****
DAIRY PRODUCTS	Note high fat levels in butter, whole milk and many cheeses ▼				
Butter, Lurpack spreadable, 10g (about one dessert spoon)	73	8 (3.7)	0.09	0	1

Type of food[1]	Calories	Fat grams (of which saturates)	Salt grams	Fibre grams	Sugar grams
Butter, Anchor spreadable, 10g	72	8 (3)	0.12	0	<1
Spread, Utterly Butterly, 10g	53	6 (1.5)	0.16	0	0.5
Spread, Flora original, 10g	53	6 (1.2)	0.1	0	<1
Spread, St Ivel extra light, 10g	19	2 (0.5)	0.1	0.13	0.14
Milk whole, 200 ml, 1 glass	128	7 (4.8)	0.2	0	9.4
Milk semi-skimmed, 200 ml	100	3.6 (2.2)	0.2	0	9.6
Milk skimmed, 200 ml	73	0.6 (0.2)	0.2	0	9.8
Milk, chocolate flavour, Superlife, 200 ml	126	1.2 (0.8)	0.25	1	20.8 *
Milk Soya, organic, unsweetened, 200 ml	65	3.8 (0.6)	0	1.2	0.2

Yoghurt natural Greek style, 100g (3.5oz)	145	11 (7)*	0.3	0	6.6
Yoghurt natural, low fat, 100g (3.5oz)	65	1.5 (0.9)	0.2	0	7.2
Yoghurt Muller Light cherry, 100g	48	0.1 (0.1)	0.1	0.2	6.4
Yoghurt Muller Light strawberry, 100g	51	0.1 (0.1)	0.1	0.2	7.2
Cheese, Brie, 100g	334	28 (17)*	0.6	0	0.45
Cheese, Brie healthy, 100g	60	3.3 (2)	0.5	0	0
Cheese, Camambert, average all brands, 100g	300	24 (15.3)	2.1	0	0.6
Cheese, Cheddar extra mature, West Country Farmhouse, 100g	412	34 (23)*	1.75	0	0
Cheese, Danish Blue, 100g	350	29 (18.3)	3.7	0	0.7

Cheese, Dutch Edam, 100g	335	25 (17)**	2.6	0	0.1
Cheese, Natural Cottage, 100g	105	4.8 (2.3)	0.75	0.6	1.8
Cheese, Parmesan, grated, 100g, ca. 1 cup	431	28.6 (17.3)*	1.5	0	0.9
Cheese, Wegmans, Stilton, white with apricots, 100g	333	26.7 (20)	1.75	3.3	10
Cheese spread, Kraft Philadelphia, one tablespoon, ca. 30g	75	7.2 (4.8)	0.25	0	1
Cheese spread, Kraft Philadephia Light, 30g	47	3.5 (2.3)	0.75	0.1	1.2
Eggs, 1 egg, 55g	83	$6.2 (1.8)^3$	0.1	0	0
Eggs, 2 scrambled, variable depends if use skimmed or whole milk	200 +	14+ (4+) cholesterol	0.5	0	1.4

CEREALS/CEREAL PRODUCTS – FLOUR, RICE, BREADS, BREAKFAST CEREALS ETC	Note high salt levels in one slice of some bread and high salt and sugar levels in many cereals. ▼ ▽				
Type of food[1]	Calories	Fat grams (of which saturates)	Salt grams	Fibre grams	Sugar grams
Flour, McDougalls, self raising, 100g	315	1.4 (0.2)	0.75	3	1.3
Flour, Allinson, self raising, whole meal, 100g	325	2.2 (0.4)	0.75	9	1.9
Pasta, Penne, white, dry, 100g	357	1.7 (0.5)	0.3	2.5	3.5
Pasta, Penne, wholemeal, dry, 100g	316	2 (0.4)	0.3	10	4
Rice, Uncle Bens, long grain, raw, 100g	344	1.25	0	1	0.5

Rice, Ambrosia, creamy rice pudding, tinned, 200g	186	3.6 (2.2)	0.5	0	16.4
Rice, Ambrosia, low fat rice pudding, tinned, 200g	166	1.6 (0.8)	0.5	0	16.4
Bagels,New York,plain white,1 bagel(85g)	216	1.6 (0.2)	0.7	2.5	5.1
Bagels, Food Doctor, highbran + seed + cranberry, 1 bagel	212	1.6 (0.34)	0.5	5.7	7.14
Bread, Kingsmill soft white, 1 slice	111	1.2 (0.1)	0.55	1.2	1.9
Bread, Kingsmill, wholemeal, 1 thick slice	100	1.7 (0.2)	0.46	2.7	1.9
Bread, Tesco, white, 1 thick slice	105	0.7 (0.1)	0.5	1.3	1.9
Bread, Tesco, organic white, 1 thick slice	110	1 (0.1)	0.5	1.4	1.4

Bread, Hovis, square cut white, 1 extra thick slice	155	1 (0)	1**	2	3
Bread, Hovis, organic, wholemeal, 1 slice	92	1.3	0.48	3.3	1.6
Bread, Nimble, white, 1 slice (ca.20g)	49	0.4	0.28	0.4	9.3?
Bread, Nimble, wholemeal, 1 slice	48	0.6 (0.1)	0.23	1.5	0.5
Bread, Warburtons, Danish lighter white, 1 slice (26g)	61	0.4 (0.2)	0.3	0.6	0.6
Bread, Master-macher, organic sunflower seed wholemeal rye, 100g	191	3.6 (0.6)	1.25	7.9	0.7
Bread, malt loaf, Tesco, 1 x 30g slice	81	0.48 (0.24)	0.24	6.2	1.86
Bread, garlic, Tesco, 2 white baguettes, ½ baguette	300	15.9 (9.9)**	0.8	2	2

Bread, Naan, ½ naan bread	269	11 (?)	trace	1.7	40? carbs
Poppadoms, Sainsbury, plain, fried in vegetable oil, 3 = 24g	96	4.2 (?)	0	2.1	10.2 ? carbs
Croissant, Tesco Healthy Living, 1 croissant, 48g	153	4.1 (2.4)	0.5	1.6	3
Croissant, Tesco Finest, all butter, 1 croissant	330	19.4 (11.7)**	0.75	1.7	3
Cereal bars, Tesco, fruit and fibre, 1 bar, 27g	110	2.7 (1.1)	0.25	1.1	7.3
Cereal bars, Jordans, special muesli, 1 bar, 40g	151	4.6 (1.2)	trace	2.3	15.6
Cereal bars, Kellogg's, nutri-grain, choc-chip, 1 bar, 45g	179	6 (1.5)	0.2	1.5	16
Hot cross buns, Tesco Finest, white, 1 bun	205	3.2 (1.4)	0.5	2.3	13.5

All Bran, Kellogg's, 100g	280	3.5 (0.7)	1.5	27	17
Branflakes, Tesco, 100g	326	2 (0.5)	1.3	15	22
Coco Pops, Kellogg's, 100g	387	3 (1.5)	1.15	2	36 ***
Cornflakes, Kellogg's, 100g (3.5oz)	372	0.9 (0.2)	1.8**	3	8
Cornflakes, Tesco, 100g	380	1.2 (0.4)	0.6	3	8.9
Cornflakes Crunchy Nut, Kellogg's, 100g	397	5 (0.9)	1.15	2.5	35***
Frosties, Kellogg's, 100g (3.5oz)	371	0.6 (0.1)	1.15	2	37**
Fruit and Fibre, Tesco, 100g (3.5oz)	370	6.6 (3.6)	0.75	7.7	26.5 **
Oatibix, Weetabix, 2 biscuits	181	3.8 (0.6)	0.18	3.5	1.5
Special K, Kellogg's, 100g	374	1.5 (0.5)	1.15	2.5	17

Shredded Wheat, Nestle, 2 biscuits, 44g	217	3.2 (1.4)	0	5.3	6.3
Weetabix, 2 biscuits, 38g	127	0.75	0.24	3.75	4.4
Muesli, Alpen Original, 100g	359	5.8 (0.7)	0.38	7.3	22*
Muesli, Alpen no added sugar, 100g	353	5.9 (0.7)	0.43	7.7	16
Muesli, Tesco Swiss Style, 100g	359	5.3 (0.8)	0.5	7.4	21*
Porridge, Tesco, organic, 100g	360	8.1 (1.6)	0	8.5	1.5
Porridge, Scots Porridge Oats, original, 100g	356	8 (1.5)	0	9	1.1
Porridge, Ready Brek, 100g	359	8.7 (1.2)	trace	7.9	1

VEGETABLES, FRUITS AND NUTS	This list is not exhaustive since most vegetables and fruit are low in calories, harmful fat, salt, and sugar as well as containing beneficial fibre				
	▼	▼	▼	▼	▼
Beans, fine green, organic, 100g (3.5oz)	25	0.5	0	-	2.3
Broccoli, 100g (3.5oz)	31	0.2	0	2.7	1.1
Broad beans, baby, frozen, 100g	72	0.9	0	4.6	0.9
Butter beans, raw, 100g	305	1.7 (0.2)	0	16	3.6
Carrots, 100g	36	0.3	0	2.5	7.4
Peas, frozen, 100g	77	0.25	0	5.5	4.6
Peppers, organic, 1 pepper	11	0.2	0	-	9
Potato, baking, 1 potato, ca. 175g	138	0.4	0	2.3	1.1

Salad, Tesco French style crispy, 40g	6	0.2	0	0.6	0.6
Stir-fry, Tesco vegetables, 100g	31	0.4	0	2.6	4.5
Sweetcorn, 100g	110	2.3 (0.3)	0	2.8	2.2
Tomatoes, Tesco, Italian, peeled, plum, 200g = half can	46	0.4	0	1.8	8
Apples, Granny Smith, 1 apple, ca. 133g	64	0	0	2.3	15.2 [4]
Avocado, 1 ca. 145g	275	28.3 (5.9)[5]	0	4.9	0.7
Banana, 1 medium size	119	0.4 (0.1)	0	1	26[4]
Blueberries, 3 heaped table-spoons, ca.50g	25	0.2	0	1.4	5.5

Type of food[1]	Calories	Fat grams (of which saturates)	Salt grams	Fibre grams	Sugar grams
Grapes, red seedless, 10 grapes, ca. 50g	30	0	0	0.35	7.7
Mango, 250g	143	0.5	0	6.5	34.5 [4]
Melon, honeydew, 1 cup, balls, 177g	64	0.2	0.1	1.4	14.4 [4]
Oranges, 1 ca. 154g, edible part	59	0.2	0	2.6	13.1 [4]
Pears, 1 ca. 170g	68	0.1	0	3.7	26[4]
Pumpkin seeds, Neal's Yard, organic,15g	85	6.6 (1)	trace	0.8	0.16
Sultanas, Neal's Yard, organic, per 15g	42	trace	trace	0.3	10.4 [4]
Tinned prunes in fruit juice, ½ can, ca. 90g	125	0.3	0	3.5	28.6 [4]

Tinned prunes in syrup, ½ can, ca. 120g	205	0.4	0	5.9	48.3 **
Pineapple, 100g	44	0.2	0	1.2	10.1
Strawberries, organic, 100g (3.5oz)	27	0.1	0	1.1	6
Brazil nuts, Planters, 50g, about 12 nuts	339	34 (7.1)[5]	0	3.6	1.8
Peanuts, dry roasted, KP, 1 small bag, 50g	292	23.1 (4)[5]	1	3.3	2.6
Peanuts, original salted, KP , 1 small bag, 50g	295	24.5 (4.4)[5]	0.75	4.5	2.7
Walnuts, Planters, 50g	375	35.7 (3.5)[5]	trace	3.5	1.8

READY MEALS, PASTAS, PIZZAS, ⬜QUICHES	Note that many of these are very high in calories, fat, salt and sugar. Compare also Tesco Healthy Living Options with Tesco Finest (Finest Fat Levels*) ▼		▼	▼		▼
MOST OF THE MEALS BELOW ARE SOLD FOR EATING JUST BY ONE PERSON AND THEREFORE DATA ARE SHOWN FOR THE **WHOLE MEAL** RATHER THAN PER 100G						
Chicken tikka masala and rice, Tesco Healthy Living, 450g	480	8.6 (2.6)	1.1	3.6		13.8
Chicken tikka masala and rice, Tesco Finest, 375g	510	35.9 (13.7) **	2.4	5.7		10.5
Chicken korma and rice, Tesco Healthy Living, 450g	487	9.9 (5)	1.3	3.5	11.3	
Chicken korma and rice, Tesco Finest, 500g	830 ****	45 (16.6) **	2.9	4.7		9.3

87

Chicken mango curry and rice, Tesco Healthy Living, 450g	495	8.1 (3.1)	1.7	4.1	20.3 **
Vegetarian vegetable korma and rice, Tesco, 450g	621 **	26.4 (10.2) **	2.2	6.3	17.6
Beef and black bean sauce, Tesco Finest, 350g	336	10.9 (2.3)	3.3	5.7	16.2
Sweet and sour chicken, Tesco Finest, 400g	560	16 (2.2)	3.2	3.4	37.8 ***
Cannelloni, beef, Tesco Finest, 400g	545	30.5 (11.6)**	2.1	4.5	11.7
Chicken with mozzarella & pancetta, Tesco Finest, 450g	830	50.2 (28.2) ***	3	7.4	1

Cornbeef hash, Tesco frozen, 400g	500	17.4 (9.2)	3.6	5	0.2
Cottage pie, Tesco Healthy Living, 500g	460	13.2 (7)	1.9	5.2	2.8
Fish pie, creamy, Tesco Finest, 400g	500	26.5 (13.9)	2.1	5.3	4.4
Lasagne, Tesco Finest, 620g	850	44.6 (21)***	3.8	5	1.2
Lasagne, Tesco Healthy Living, 430g	426	11.2 (5.6)	2.3	3	1.7
Macaroni cheese, Tesco Healthy Living, 385g	420	8.9 (6)	1.7	5.8	8.9
Moussaka, lamb, Tesco Finest, 350g	510	38 (8.2)**	2	12	11.9
Pasta bake, chicken, Tesco Healthy Living, 400g	415	5.6 (2.9)	1	5.6	7.2
Pasta bake, tuna, Tesco Healthy Living, 400g	360	4.4 (1.9)	1.5	4.4	9.6

Pasta, cheese, Tesco, 400g	940***	63 (16.4)***	1.2	3.2	7.2
Pasta, tomato, Tesco, 400g	760	36 (2.8)	4.5	5.6	18
Pizza, cheese, Tesco, 395g, ½	495	17.6 (7.1)	2.8	7.5	4.5
Pizza, ham + **pineapple,** Tesco, 466g, ½	480	14.9 (6.5)	2.2	6.8	11.2
Pizza, pepperoni, Tesco, 398g, ½	510	18.7 (6.4)	3.1	5.6	4.6
Pizza, pizzeria, **margherita,** Tesco, 460g, ½	545	24.4 (12.9)**	2.2	6.2	4.8
Quiche, cheese and **bacon,** Tesco, 330g, ½	460	30.8 (12.4)**	1.2	2	4.8
Quiche, cheese and **onion,** 330g, ½	460	30.2 (12.8)**	1	1.8	5.6
Strogonoff, **vegetarian,** **mushroom,** Tesco, 450g	526	21.9 (13.2)**	1.5	5.5	4.3

SALADS, DIPS AND SANDWICHES	Note high calorie, saturated fat and salt levels in some items especially sandwiches ▼ ▼ ▼				
Salad, chicken layered bowl, 200g	135	1 (0.2)	0.5	4	4.8
Salad, chicken and bacon, layered bowl, 200g	247	13.4 (1.2)	0.5	4	4.8
Salad, cheese layered bowl, 200g	335	26.4 (6.6)	0.7	3.2	5.8
Salad, prawn layered bowl, 200g	270	17.2 (2.5)	1.1	2.4	3.2
Salad, tuna layered bowl, 200g	274	14.2 (0.9)	0.2	2.9	3.7
Salad, creamy coleslaw and potato, 200g	450	45 (4.4)	1	3	4.3
Dip, caramelized onion & roast garlic, ¼ pot, 50g	250	26 (3.4)	0.6	0.2	1.6

Dip, caramelized onion humous, reduced fat, ¼ pot, 50g	79	4.5 (0.5)	0.6	-	2.8
Dip, cheese and chive, ¼ pot, 50g	270	27.4 (4.2)	0.6	-	1
Dip, guacamole, ¼ pot, 50g	105	10.5 (4)	0.3	1.8	0.9
Dip, humous, ¼ pot, 50g	160	13.4 (1.4)	0.7	1.7	0.5
Dip, salsa, ¼ pot, 50g	28	1.2	0.6	0.6	2.8
Dip, sour cream & chives, ¼ pot, 50g	180	18.4 (4.2)	0.4	-	1.2
Dip, West Country Cheddar, ¼ pot, 50g	255	25.9 (4.19)	0.6	0	1.19
Make your own low fat sandwiches - see [6]					
Sandwiches, Pret a Manger, all day breakfast, malted wholegrain, 2 sandwiches	608	35.7 (8.6)**	3.54*	4.2	8

Sandwiches, cheese and chutney, with mayo, organic, malted brown, 2 sandwiches	545	29.2 (14) **	2.1	5.2	11.2
Sandwiches, cheese and onion, with mayo, brown + oatmeal, 2 sandwiches	555	33.1 (12.1) **	1.8	5.5	3.5
Sandwiches, chicken salad, malted brown, 2 sandwiches	445	20 (3.7)	1.2	6.3	4.3
Sandwiches, chicken and bacon, sub roll, white	645	29.1 (3.6)**	2	5.2	7.2
Sandwiches, ploughman's, wedge, white	605	32 (13.8)**	2.3	5.4	13.8
Sandwiches, prawn & mayo, white + oatmeal, 2 sandwiches	430	25.7	1.75	4	2.5

Sandwiches, red Chedder and tomato, white, 2 sandwiches	490	26.6 (10.5)**	2.2	5.5	2.9
Sandwiches, roast beef, Tesco Finest, malted brown, 2 sandwiches	450	17.1 (4.6)	2.9*	ca.4 .6	8.2
Sandwiches, salmon & cucumber, Tesco Healthy Living, 2 sandwiches	262	4 (0.9)	1.5	3.3	2.6
Sandwiches, smoked ham & mustard, white, 2 sandwiches	385	16.8 (3.6)	2.9*	1.9	5.9
Sandwiches, tuna-sweetcorn, malted brown, 2 sandwiches	440	21.1 (3.5)	2.5	4.4	4

Type of food[1]	Calories	Fat grams (of which satu-rates)	Salt grams	Fibre grams	Sugar grams
SNACKS-BISCUITS, CAKES, CHOCOLATE AND ICE-CREAM	Note that many of these are very high in calories, fat, salt and sugar. These are really harmful snacks if eaten in excess daily. We all have to eat some occasionally! ▼	▼	▼		▼
Biscuits, Mcvitie's milk chocolate digestive, 4 biscuits	336	16 (8.4)**	1	2	20**
Biscuits, Mcvitie's original digestive, 4 biscuits	280	13 (6)	1	2	10
Biscuits, Mcvitie's chocolate chip cookies, 4 biscuits	332	18 (10)**	1	2.4	22.4**
Biscuits, Mcvitie's Hobnobs, 4 biscuits	268	12.4 (5.6)	1	3.2	13.6
Biscuits, Mcvitie's Hobnob flapjacks, 1 flapjack, 33g	313	14.6 (6.5)	0.5	4.7	20.5**

Biscuits, Mcvitie's Penguins, 2 biscuits	228	12.2 (7.8)*	trace	1	17.8*
Biscuits, Jammie Dodgers, 4 biscuits	332	12 (5.6)	trace	1.6	22.4**
Biscuits, Cadbury's chocolate fingers, 8 Fingers	240	12 (4.8)	trace	0.8	15.2
Biscuits, Jacob's fig rolls, 4 biscuits	252	6 (2.8)	<1	2.4	21.6**
Biscuits, Mcvitie's classic rich tea, 4 biscuits	152	5.2 (2)	<1	0.8	6.8
Biscuits, Tesco, Custard Creams, 4 biscuits	240	10.4 (6.4)	0.1	0.8	12.8
Biscuits, Cookie Coach, clotted cream shortbread fingers, 4 fingers	424*	24.2**	?	?	46.4** carbs

Biscuits, Jaffa Cakes, 4 biscuits	184	4 (2)	trace	1.2	26**
Cakes, doughnut, fresh cream, one	260	12.6 (6.4)	0.6	1.5	11.6
Cakes, cheesecake, strawberry and double cream, $^1/_5$, 100g	271	13.4 (6.6)	0.2	1.6	22**
Cakes, Cupcakes, Bakin Boys, triple chocolate, one	156	9 (3)	0.1	1	12
Chocolate, Aero, 46g bar	251	14.5 (9.4)**	0.1	0.4	26.8**
Chocolate, Bounty Milk, 57g bar	267	6.8 (?)	0.14	1.2	13.6
Chocolate, Cadbury's Dairy Milk, 10 squares = 40g	220	12 (8)**	0.1	1	21**
Chocolate, Cadbury's, Dairy Milk, whole nut, 49g bar	270	17.3 (8)**	0.1	?	23.6**

Chocolate, Galaxy bar, milk chocolate, 47g bar	254	14.8 (?)	?	?	27.1 Carbs
Chocolate, Kit Kat, 4 finger bar, 42g	212	11(?)	?	0	26 Carbs
Chocolate, Maltesers, one bag, 37g	183	8.5 (?)	?	0	24 carbs
Chocolate, Mars bar, 65g bar	284	11.1 (ca.6.5)	?	0	45** carbs
Chocolate, M&Ms, peanut chocolate candies, 45g bag	232	11.7 (4.7)	?	1.5	22.9**
Chocolate, Plain, Tesco, 50g (1.75oz)	259	13.5 (8.5)**	0	1.6	29.2**
Chocolate, Plain, Marks and Spencer, extra fine dark chocolate 50g	277	22.6 (13.6) **	0	6	13.5

Chocolate, Snickers, 62.5g bar	319	17.8 (ca.6.4)	0.35	1	ca.30 **
Chocolate, Twix, two fingers, 57g	284	13.9 (5.1)	0.28	0.6	27.4**
Ice-cream, cherrylicious, Tesco, 200 ml serving, about 2 scoops	240	6.8 (5.8)	trace	1	22.6**
Ice-cream, Cornish, Walls, 200 ml	166	8 (5.4)	0.26	0.2	18.4
Ice-cream, vanilla, Carte D'Or, 200 ml	240	11 (?)	?	?	29 carbs*
SNACKS-TINNED BEANS AND SPAGHETTI, CHIPS, CRISPS AND ⬚ SOUPS	Note that some items are high in calories and fat but that healthier options do exist ▼ ▼				
Beans, baked and tinned, Heinz, 100g	73	0.2 (trace)	0.8	3.8	5

Beans, baked and tinned, Heinz, reduced sugar and salt, 100g	66	0.2 (trace)	0.5	3.8	3.4
Spaghetti, tinned, Heinz, 100g	60	0.3 (trace)	0.6	2.4	4
Chips, Tesco oven chips, crinkle cut, 100g (3.5oz)	140	3.9 (0.5)	0.2	1.8	<0.1
Chips, McDonald's, medium portion	340	17 (2)	0.7	4	1
Chips, Burger King, french fries, medium portion, 117g	387	20 (5)*	1.3	3	1
Crisps, Doritos, cool original, 40g pack	200	11 (1)	0.8	1.2	1.6[7]
Crisps, Hula Hoops, salt and vinegar, 34g pack	174	9.7 (0.9)	0.75	0.6	0.3[7]
Crisps, McCoy's, ridge cut, salted, 50g pack	262	16 (4.8)	1	2.1	0.2

Crisps, McCoy's, ridge cut, cheddar and onion, 50g pack	258	15.3 (4.6)	1	2	1[7]
Crisps, McCoy's, ridge cut, salt and vinegar, 50g	257	3.1 (2)[7L]	1.4	2	0.5[7]
Crisps, Walkers, prawn cocktail, 34.5g pack	181	11.4 (0.9)	0.5	1.4	0.7[7]
Crisps, Walkers, ready salted, 34.5g pack	183	11.7 (0.9)	0.5	1.4	0.3
Crisps, Walkers, cheese and onion, 25g pack	131	8.3 (0.7)	0.32	1	0.6[7]
Soup, cream of tomato, ½ can, 300g,	169	5.7 (1.1)	1.6	1.2	15.5
Soup, chicken and sweetcorn, ½ can, 300g	127	2.7 (1.4)	1.1	2.4	5.7
Soup, pea and ham, ½ can, 300g	164	6.3 (3.9)	1.4	3.6	8

SNACKS-FISH FINGERS, KEBABS, PIES, PASTIES, RIBS, SAUSAGE ☐ ROLLS, AND WINGS	Not surprisingly many of these items are high in calories and fat ▼ ▼			
Fish fingers, Tesco "Free From", 3 fish fingers, 90g	180	8.1 (3.9)	0.9	0.6	trace
Kebabs, Tesco, 12 chicken tikka, pack =130g,	216	9.6 (3.6)	1.2	1.2	8.4
Pie, chicken and vegetable, each pie, 150g (5.4 oz)	390	21.8 (11.1) **	1.5	1.7	2.4
Pie, steak, 150g	445	27 (13)**	1.5	3.8	1.7
Pasty, Cornish, 150g	433	26.8 (12.7) **	1.7	5.7	3.5
Pasty, cheese, 150g	392	23.5 (11.3) **	1.7	5.8	3.4

Ribs, sticky barbecue, ½ pack, 400g	325	21.8 (9.2)**	0.7	1.9	10.5
Sausage rolls, Tesco, pack of 6, medium/large 400g, each roll 66.5g	240	16.2 (7.1)**	1	0.7	0.5
Wings, sticky barbecue chicken, ¼ pack of 500g	180	10.6 (2.8)	0.8	0.5	2.9
DRINKS-SOFT, JUICES, BED-TIME, ▶ COFFEE, TEA AND ALCOHOL ▼	The items causing the main concern here are added sugar in soft and bed-time drinks and the high calories in bed-time and alcoholic drinks. ▼				
Soft drink, Coca Cola, 250 ml glass, sugar added	105	0	0	0	27[7] *
Soft drink, Diet Coca Cola, 250 ml glass	3.5	0	0	0	0[8]
Soft drink, Ribena, blackcurrant, from concentrate, 250 ml glass + added sugar	128	0	0	0	30.3*

Soft drink, Juiceburst, pomegranate, from concentrate, 250 ml + added sugar	122	<0.25	?	?	28.75 *
Soft drink, Fanta orange, 250 ml glass, added sugar	108	0	trace	0	26.3*[7]
Soft drink, lemonade, 250 ml glass, added sugar	117	0	0	0	28.5*
Soft drink, Robinsons orange barley water, diluted 45 ml in 250 ml glass	45	0	0.025	0	9
Fruit juice, apple, Sainsbury, from concentrate, 250 ml glass	117	<0.12	<0.4	<0.12	28[9]
Fruit juice, cranberry, Sainsbury, from 10% concentrate, 250 ml glass + added sugar	123	trace	trace	trace	29.8*

Fruit juice, orange, Sainsbury, 100% pure squeezed, 250 ml glass	110	0	<0.3	1	24.2^9
Fruit juice, pineapple, Sainsbury, pure from concentrate, 250 ml glass	132	<0.12	<0.4	<0.12	31^9
Fruit juice, pomegranate, RJA Foods, superjuice, from concentrate, 250 ml glass	110	<0.1	trace	0	26.5??
Fruit juice, tomato, Sainsbury, from concentrate, 250 ml glass	37	<0.12	2	1.7	6.7
Bed-time drink, Bournville Cocoa, Cadbury, per 4g with semi-skimmed milk	110	4.3 (2.5)	0.35	0.5	10^9

Bed-time drink, Bournvita, Cadbury, per 12g serving	140	3.7(?)	?	?	20[9] carbs
Bed-time drink, instant hot chocolate, Tesco, 30g in water	125	3 (2.6)	0.5	0.6	19.1
Bed-time drink, Horlicks original, per 20g with 200 ml semi-skimmed milk	186	4.6 (2.6)	0.5	0.7	19.6
Bed-time drink, Ovaltine original, per 25g with semi-skimmed milk	187	3.8 (2.1)	0.4	0.6	21.71 *
Bed-time drink, Ovaltine original light, per 25g in water	90	1.5 (0.9)	0.25	0.75	14
Coffee, black, brewed/instant, 240 ml cup	12/6	0	trace	0	0
Coffee, cappuccino, Starbucks, with skimmed milk, 240 ml cup	52	0	0.17	0	6.4

Coffee, cappuccino, Starbucks, with whole milk, 240 ml cup	84	4.4 (2.8)	0.16	0	6
Coffee, espresso, Starbucks, 30 ml single	5	0	0	0	0
Coffee, espresso, Starbucks, 30 ml single shot + dollop whipped cream	110	9 (6)*	0.02	0	2
Coffee, latte, Starbucks, with skimmed milk, 240 ml cup	84	0	0.29	0	10
Coffee, latte, Starbucks, with whole milk, 240 ml cup	136	7 (4.4)	0.26	0	9.6
Coffee-mate, Nestle, per 6.5g teaspoon	36	2.2 (2.2) 10	0.1	0	0.6
Teas, ordinary brands, no milk or sugar, 240 ml cup	0	0	0	0	0

Teas, ordinary brands, with 30 ml semi-skimmed milk and 5g (1 teaspoon) sugar	34	0.5 (0.3)	trace	0	5
Alcohol, beer, bitter, 1 pint (568 ml)	182	0	trace	0	20 carbs
Alcohol, beer, Buweiser, 1 pint	183	0	trace	0	0
Alcohol, beer, Guiness, 1 pint	170	0	trace	0	8.5 carbs
Alcohol, beer, lager, Stella, 1 pint	229	0	trace	0	16 carbs
Alcohol, champagne, 120 ml glass	91	0	trace	0	1.7 carbs
Alcohol, gin, 40%, double, 50 ml	112	0	0	0	0
Alcohol, vodka, 40%, double, 50 ml	110	0	0	0	0
Alcohol, white wine, 120 ml glass	89	0	trace	0	3.6 carbs

Alcohol, whiskey, 40%, double, 50 ml	107	0	0	0	0
Alcohol, wine **red, Burgundy,** 120 ml glass	104	0	trace	0	4.4 carbs
DRESSINGS, PICKLES, SAUCES, GRAVIES, SPREADS ⬚ **AND JAMS**	Many items are high in calories and salt but healthier options are available ▼ ▼				
Dressing, Real Mayonnaise, Hellmann's, per 20g serving	145	15.8 (1.3)	0.3	0	0.3
Dressing, Light Mayonnaise, Hellmann's, per 20g	59	6 (0.6)	0.46	0	0.4
Dressing, Salad Cream, Heinz, per 20g	66	5.4 (0.6)	0.5	trace	3.5

Type of food[1]	Calories	Fat grams (of which saturates)	Salt grams	Fibre grams	Sugar grams
Dressing, fat-free vinaigrette, Hellmann's, per 20 ml	47	0	0.18	trace	2.2
Dressing, French vinaigrette, Tesco Finest, 20 ml	92	8 (0.8)	0.3	0.1	1.1
Dressing, Italian, Newman's Own, per 20g	109	12 (?)	0.4	?	1 carbs
Pickle, original pickle, Branston, 1 tablespoon, 15g	16	trace	0.6	0.2	3.6
Pickle, original Picalli, Tesco, 15g	12	trace	0.3	0.2	2.4
Pickle, olives in brine, whole green, 15g	20	2 (0.4)	0.8	3.1	trace

Pickle onions in sweet vinegar, Sainsbury, excess vinegar dried, per 15g	5	trace	0.26	1.1	0.9
Sauce, tomato ketchup, Heinz, per 20g	20	trace	0.6	0.1	4.7
Sauce, brown, HP original, per 20g	24	trace	0.5	0.3	4.5
Sauce, pasta, slow roasted garlic and chilli, Seeds of Chang organic, 100g	73	4.5 (1.3)	1.4	1	7.3
Sauce, pasta, tomato and basil, Seeds of Change, organic, 100g	59	2 (0.4)	0.8	0.8	7.8
Sauce, pasta, traditional bolognaise Seeds Of Change, organic,100g	58	1.2 (0.3)	1	0.8	8.9
Sauce cooking, Indian, Korma, Sherwoods, gluten – free, 100g	136	7.8 (4.4)	1	2.2	7.7

Sauce cooking, Indian, Rogan Josh, Sherwoods, 100g	71	3.8 (0.3)	1	3.5	4.7
Sauce cooking, Indian, Tikka Masala, Sherwoods, 100g	116	7.7 (3.3)	1.6	1.6	6
Sauce cooking, Chinese, black bean and red pepper, Sherwoods, 100g	62	1.4 (0.2)	1.7	1.2	5.9
Sauce cooking, Chinese, sweet and sour, Sherwoods, 100g	105	0.5 (trace)	0.9	0.8	17.9
Gravy, Oxo beef, each cube, 5.9g	16	0.27 (0.13)	2.5	trace	0.15
Gravy, Bisto original, 4 level teaspoons = 1 serving + water	9	trace	0.8	trace	0.2
Gravy, Tesco beefy drink/stock, like Bovril, 1 teaspoon	24	trace	1.4	?	trace

Spread, honey, Sainsbury, pre-set blended, 1 tablespoon, 15g	51	trace	trace	trace	13
Spread, Marmite, 4g	37	trace	0.5	0.1	trace
Spread, peanut butter, smooth, with 1 tablespoon = 15g	90	7.8 (1.5)	0.19	0.9	1.17
Jam, apricot spread, Weight Watchers, 20g	23	trace	trace	0.13	5.3
Jam, blackcurrant, reduced sugar, Sainsbury, per teaspoon	29	<0.1	<0.1	0.2	5.9
Jam, marmalade, Frank Cooper's Oxford original, coarse cut, 20g serving	54	0	0.05	0.2	11.9
Jam, raspberry, Robertsons, 20g	49	trace	<0.1	0.3	11.9
Jam, strawberry conserve, Tesco Finest, 20g	50	trace	trace	0.2	12

Remember, stars in dark grey boxes indicate very high levels of calories, fat, salt or sugar. Often, calories, fat etc are given per 100g of food item but servings actually eaten, as with cheese, are much less than this.

1. Unless otherwise indicated, the data for many food items were taken from Tesco supermarkets.

2. Whenever possible, not only fat but also saturated fat levels are given in brackets.

Saturated fats raise bad cholesterol in the blood and can lead to heart disease and other health problems (see Chapter 3 "Fats – the Good, the Bad and the Ugly").

3. Eggs are packed with protein, vitamins and minerals and have been called a superfood. The yolk, however, does have high cholesterol levels but one egg a day is unlikely to affect cholesterol level in the blood and increase heart disease (see reference 11).

4. Many fruits such as apples, bananas, mangoes, and pears, have a high sugar content but these natural sugars (called fructose) in fruit and vegetables are beneficial and different to sugar (sucrose) added to our food. Fructose is broken down slowly by the body and does not cause a sudden increase in blood sugar. In contrast, sucrose added to food causes a sudden rapid increase in blood sugar (sucrose is rapidly broken down to glucose=blood sugar) and overworks the pancreas to release insulin. Too many sudden increases in blood glucose from sucrose can stress the pancreas and may potentially lead to diabetes as well as to the conversion of the excess glucose to fat.

5. Avocados and nuts contain high levels of fat but most of this fat is monosaturated which is "good" fat and this will help reduce cholesterol.

6. See "Top tips for a healthier lunchbox" at:
www.food.gov.uk/news/newsarchive/2004/sep/lunchbox

7. These foods may contain saccharin, colourings, preservatives, stabilizers, monosodium glutamate, and/or flavourings etc. Generally, the crisps just with salt added are free of these additives. 7L= lower fat or "light" crisps are now available in many flavours.

8. Items with no added sugar but with artificial sweeteners (aspartame), flavourings, colourings, citric and phosphoric acids etc.

9. These have no added sugar and contain only natural sugar from the fruit-see 4 above.

10. Contains hydrogenated vegetable oils.

CHANGES IN DIET WITH AGE

A FACT OF LIFE! As you age, your metabolism slows down, you have less energy and so you need fewer calories. Unless you eat fewer calories or become more active, you will slowly gain weight and gradually fat will accumulate to eventually form a bulging stomach, backside, legs, arms and face which will result in becoming overweight and eventually possibly obesity too. These changes are particularly marked by an increase in waist measurement and in the size of clothes worn-the so-called "**middle age spread**". These changes are not inevitable as explained in detail in reference 12.

REALISE THAT FAT AND WEIGHT WILL ACCUMULATE WHEN:

"CALORIES EATEN EXCEED CALORIES USED BY BODY"

There are **TWO OPTIONS** to avoid weight gain with age:

1. **Reduce calorie intake** by gradually changing your diet such as switching to skimmed milk and avoiding high fat snacks (see Chapter 11 of IYL, Table 2).

2. **Increase calories burnt** by slowly increasing the amount or frequency of exercise. This will not only burn the excess calories but also increase your muscular mass and metabolic rate. **MOST IMPORTANT TOO** is that age-related muscle wasting (Sarcopenia) will also be avoided and the ability to live independently will be retained longer (see Chapter 11 of IYL, pages 217-220).

The reduced metabolism with age results from the loss of muscle mass and an increase in fat deposits. Muscles burn calories more actively than fat so any exercise to strengthen the muscles will also raise the metabolic rate. Unfortunately, since women have less muscular mass than men the reduction in the metabolic rate with age in women is more rapid than in men. **Women are therefore more prone than men to gain weight with age.**

Therefore, the calorific excesses some women inflict on their bodies, in particular, by drinking pints of lager, will probably be reflected by more rapid weight gain in women than in men.

Other dietary modifications with age. All the advice given above in this chapter about healthy eating should continue to be followed i.e.:

Table 2.   Summary of Dietary Advice

1. Eat breakfast

2. Avoid processed food and
    unhealthy snacks

3. Eat less saturated fats and
    trans fats

4. Avoid foods with too much
    salt added

5. Eat plenty of fruit and
    vegetables

6. Have a enough fibre and
    water each day

7. Read and understand food
    labels

IN ADDITION, other changes gradually occur as we age that will affect our nutrition:

- Retirement may restrict the money available for food

- Death of, or separation from, partner may result in depression and poorly prepared food

- Senses such as sight, taste and smell of food will diminish and reduce interest in food

- Our ability to absorb certain key nutrients may be reduced sometimes as a result of medicines taken

- Constipation may be common due a reduction in saliva production and slower movements of food through the gut

- Neglect of the teeth and oral hygiene may result in inclusion of softer and more processed rather than fresh food in the diet

- **IT ALL SOUNDS VERY DEPRESSING** but remember the 7 points listed about diet (above, Table 2) as well as the following advice in Figure 1 and Table 3 (below) and sensible nutrition can then be maintained.

Figure 1. Summary points for maintaining healthy nutrition with aging[a]

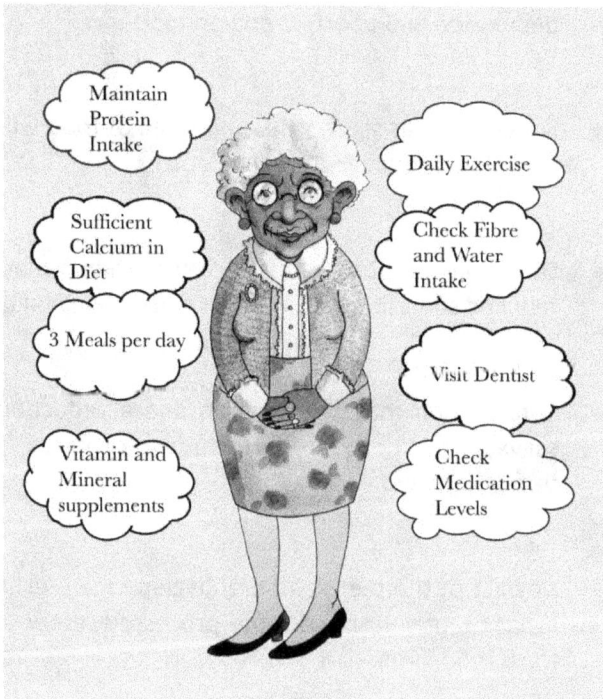

Table 3. More Details of Points in Figure 1. (above)

1. Maintain regular daily exercise to reduce depression and stimulate the appetite, to meet friends, and to maintain muscular tone and healthy bones.
2. Eat three regular meals per day
3. Vary choice of food. Ensure that protein levels are high by eating sufficient lean meat, fish, low fat dairy products, beans and peas, wholemeal bread and, if possible, a whey protein drink.

4. To maintain healthy bones, make sure that sufficient sources of calcium are included in the diet. Natural calcium sources are low fat dairy products, sardines, salmon, green vegetables etc.

5. Older people with poor diets or with illnesses may require vitamin and mineral supplements. Be aware that "Recommended Daily Allowances" have been calculated for younger people. Consult your doctor as supplements may interact with medicines.

6. Reduce likelihood of constipation by increasing amount of natural high fibre foods and drinking about 8 glasses of water, juice or soup daily.

7. Regularly check with doctor that medicines taken are both necessary and at the correct dose. Also, check on possible interactions of medication with absorption of essential nutrients.

8. Visit dentist regularly to maintain healthy teeth and gums

a. See, also, Chapters 7 and 8 of IYL "Vitamins, Minerals and Supplements Dilemma"

SUMMARY

Follow the above advice together with regular exercise and you will be re-vitalised and always remember to:

• BE DETERMINED TO CHANGE
• AVOID FAD DIETS
• EAT BREAKFAST
• STOP SNACKING
• SELECT HEALTHY FOODS WITH LOWER FAT AND SALT
• GET RID OF PROCESSED FOOD FROM THE DIET
• GET ENOUGH FIBRE
• EAT AT LEAST 5 PORTIONS OF VEGETABLES OR FRUIT EACH DAY
• DRINK PLENTY OF WATER
• MAKE CHANGES GRADUALLY
• LIST REASONS FOR DECLINE IN PHYSICAL ACTIVITY

Change your lifestyle slowly so that your new diet and exercise regimens become a natural part of everyday living

CHAPTER 3

More Facts About Food, Fat, Fibre And Fad Diets

FATS – THE GOOD, THE BAD AND THE UGLY

- **"Fats are bad for you".** We have all heard this so many times. Fats are reported to cause cancer, obesity and heart disease.

- **Fats, however, are essential because they:**

    i.   make up the walls of cells and tissues

    ii.   are an energy source

    iii.   form precursors of some hormones

iv.   are involved in absorption of vitamins A, D, E, and K.

- **Confused?** No wonder! The reason for the poor understanding about fats has arisen due to the fact that there are several different types of fat in our food, namely:

  i.   **monounsaturated fats**
  ii.   **polyunsaturated fats**
  iii.   **saturated fats**
  iv.   **trans fatty acids (=hydrogenated vegetable oils)**

These 4 names for the different types of fats are the ones found on **food labels.**

It is therefore important to understand that some fats are good for us while others are bad and associated with heart disease, cancer etc.

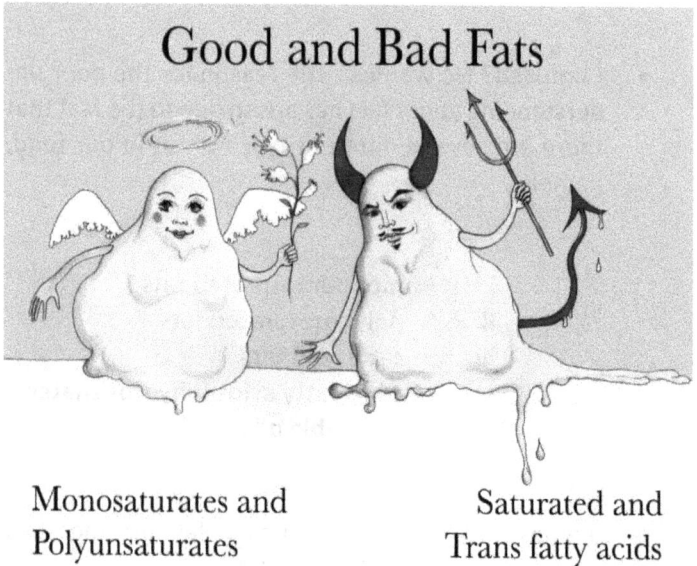

Good and Bad Fats

| Monosaturates and Polyunsaturates | Saturated and Trans fatty acids |

Good fats are the unsaturated monounsaturates and polyunsaturates. These are found mainly in vegetable oils and margarines made from these, as well as in oily fish like salmon, mackerel, sardines and pilchards (see, Table 1, below).

Bad fats are the saturated and the trans fatty acids. Saturated fats are present in full-fat dairy products, fatty meats, sausages, burgers, pies, biscuits etc. Trans fats are found in food naturally in small amounts. Most trans fats originate in the diet through "processing" by heating vegetable oils together with hydrogen. This process turns the vegetable oils semi-solid and these trans or "hydrogenated" vegetable oils are then marketed as margarines and used in biscuits, cakes, fried foods and take-way meals (see Table 1, below).

Why are some fats good and others bad? This is because the type of fat in the diet can **influence the levels of cholesterol in the blood.** High cholesterol levels are associated with increased risk of heart disease or even strokes.

You should remember 2 facts:

1. The bad fats, i.e. the saturated and trans fatty acids, **raise** the levels of cholesterol in the blood and hence increase the risk of heart disease.

2. The good fats, i.e. the monounsaturates and polyunsaturates, **reduce** the levels of harmful cholesterol in the blood and hence decrease the risk of heart disease.

Foods containing these different types of fats are summarized in Table 1:

Table 1. Showing the Distribution of Common Fats in the Diet

Type of Fat	Effect on Cholesterol Levels in Blood	Main Food Source
Monounsaturated	Lowers bad cholesterol	Olive, canola and peanut oils, most seeds and nuts (except coconuts), and avocados.
Polyunsaturated	Lowers bad cholesterol	Sunflower, corn, soybean oils or soft margarines[a.] made from these oils, oily fish such as salmon, mackerel, sardines, pilchards, trout.

Saturated	Raises bad cholesterol	Full fat dairy products such as cheese, butter, whole milk and ice cream[b], coconut and palm oils, animal fats especially red meats and poultry skin, shrimps, lard, dripping, cakes, biscuits and most savoury snacks and chocolate[c].
Trans Fatty Acids = Hydrogenated Vegetable Oils	Raises bad cholesterol	Solid or semi-solid marga-rines, some cakes, biscuits and savoury snacks as well as many deep

		fried foods such as chips, doughnuts, onion rings[d,e].

a. Check the label of soft margarine and confirm that it is free of trans fats (often labelled "hydrogenated vegetable oils" to confuse everyone) and is non-hydrogenated.

b. Skimmed milk and lower fat ice cream or some frozen yoghurts are much better.

c. It is clearly impossible to cut out all of these completely from the diet. Depending on your weight, and with moderation and exercise, some of these can still be eaten occasionally but not to excess. **Just be aware and beware of excesses** and check for dangerous trans fats.

d. These especially and c. (above) are the key foods to check in your diet as they may contain high levels of artery clogging trans fats. **Marks and Spencer has actually banned trans fats while Sainsbury's, Tesco, Co-op, Asda, and Iceland are removing from their shelves their own brand foods containing trans fats which are hydrogenated vegetable oils** (oils exposed to hydrogen to harden them at room temperature). Also, good news is that Mars, Jammie Dodgers, Wagon Wheels and McVitie's biscuits no longer contain hydrogenated oils. **Beware since some of Lidl's foods still contain these.**

e. Recently, it was reported (see reference 13) that in the UK because food companies have removed trans fats from their foods that these heart-blocking substances are well below levels causing health hazards. Huge progress has therefore been made **BUT action is still needed with food from cafes, fish bars, canteens, hospitals etc that are still using hydrogenated vegetable oils (trans fats) in food preparation.**

FINAL CONCLUSION ABOUT FATS. The bad saturated and trans fats should be reduced in the diet as this will significantly lower your risk of heart disease. Table 1 (above) is simply a guide showing which foods contain the different types of fats so that you can reduce/eliminate them from the diet. **Again modify your diet a little at a time and you will see your cholesterol levels fall as well as your excess weight.** Adopt a healthier diet as outlined above and try some regular exercise as outlined in Chapters 9-11 of IYL.

FACTS ABOUT FIBRE

- **Dietary fibre** is only found in plant and not animal products. Fibre occurs in two forms, namely, **insoluble and soluble fibre**.

- **Insoluble fibre** forms the structural support of plants, may pass straight through the gut with only minimal digestion, and helps to increase the activity of the intestine in getting rid of waste products from digestion.

- **Soluble fibre** originates from the contents of the plant cells, can be partially broken down in the gut, and absorbs water and increases the volume of faeces for ease of expulsion.

- Most fruit and vegetables contain a mixture of insoluble and soluble fibre.

- **Plant foods with high fibre levels have not been highly processed** and have not had their outer layers (seed coats etc) – which contain fibre, vitamins and minerals – removed; this removal occurs with most rice and wheat so that it is gleaming white and more attractive to the shopper.

- **Table 2 lists the fibre content of some common foods.** A balanced diet should contain about 20-25 grams of fibre per day from a mixture of fruit and vegetables (at least five per day) and high fibre breakfast cereals.

Table 2 Showing the Fibre Content of Some Common Foods[a]

Higher Levels of Fibre[b]	Lower Levels of Fibre[c]
Whole Meal Bread and Rolls	White Bread and Rolls
Whole Meal Pastas*	White Pastas**
Brown Rice	White Rice
All-Bran/Bran Flakes*	Puffed Wheat/Sugar Puffs
Weetabix*	Corn Flakes/Crunchy Nut
Shredded Wheat*	Rice Krispies, Coco Pops
Porridge Oats, Muesli	Cheerios
Baked Beans*, Peas*, Cabbage, Carrots, Spinach, Broccoli, Potatoes in skins	Salads, Tomatoes, Skinned Potatoes, Cucumber, Peppers,Celery**, Radishes

Sweetcorn	Mushrooms, Onions
Apple with skin, Pears, Avocado, Figs*, Dates, Raspberries*, Blueber-ries*, Blackberries*, Prunes*, Apricots, Oranges, Raisins and Dried Fruit* Bananas, Mangoes,	Strawberries, Grapes, Pineapples, Melons
Peanuts, Almonds* Coconuts*	Brazil Nuts, Sunflower Seeds
Yoghurts with Cereals and Berries (see which above)	Most Fruit Drinks, Plain Yoghurt

a. This Table is just a rough guide based on an average serving (100 gram or 3.5 oz) of the foods listed.

b. "High" is anything above 1.5-2 gm of fibre per serving

c. "Low" is anything below 1.5 gm of fibre per serving

    *   These foods are very high in fibre

    ** All fruits and vegetables contain some beneficial fibre. White pasta also has significant levels of fibre.

BENEFICIAL EFFECTS OF FIBRE. Health professionals commonly claim that there are many beneficial effects of sufficient fibre in the diet including reductions in:

Constipation
Diverticulitis
Irritable bowel syndrome
Cancer of colon
High cholesterol
Heart disease
Diabetes
Obesity
Gallstones

Controversy, however, does exists about the benefits of fibre. Some scientists challenge the assumption that fibre helps to prevent the above diseases.

Scientists often disagree even if the proof is beyond doubt. Unfortunately, the resulting debate once released in the media does nothing except **to confuse the public** as to what exactly they should eat. People then tend to shrug and continue with their bad habits having justified this to themselves since **"even the experts disagree"**. The inconsistent opinions over the value of fibre (and many other dietary components) often originate from the type of experimental analysis undertaken. Thus, questionnaires may be used in which people fail to make accurate returns. Alternatively, the time scale of the study may be too short and not take account of the fact that many diseases, such as cancers, may take 10-20 years or even longer to develop.

THE IMPORTANT MESSAGE ABOUT FIBRE is that it does help to keep the gut healthy by **preventing constipation** and possibly also irritable bowel syndrome, as well as the other conditions listed above. Evidence indicates that fibre is beneficial in **preventing cancer of the colon**, perhaps by speeding the expulsion or dilution of harmful toxins in the gut, or by providing anti-cancer chemicals (antioxidants, see Chapter 8 of IYL) linked to the fibre from the fruit and vegetables eaten. Fibre may also **reduce cholesterol levels**, and thus the incidence of heart disease, by binding and assisting in cholesterol excretion from the body. Fibre also slows down the rate at which glucose is absorbed from the food and prevents rapid fluctuations in blood sugar and may therefore **help to prevent and control diabetes.** Including sufficient high fibre foods in the diet may also **help control weight problems** by reducing hunger.

FINAL COMMENT AND WARNING. Adequate fibre is essential throughout life but is particularly important in **elderly people** who often have high levels of constipation. Each day in the diet include :

- Breakfast cereals with high fibre or porridge (see choice in Chapter 2 and Table 1 and Table 2 of present Chapter).

- Wholemeal bread

- Brown rice

- 5 or 6 or more portions of fruit and vegetables (peas and various types of beans have high fibre contents)

- See Table 2 of present Chapter for choice of main high fibre foods

- Drink sufficient water, milk, herbal teas, or soup to avoid dehydration with about 6-8 glasses sufficient.

- Do not sprinkle pure fibre supplements on your food as these may bind iron, calcium and zinc in your gut which will be lost down the toilet.

145

FAD OR TRENDY DIETS

COMMENTS ABOUT THE ATKINS AND GI DIETS

ATKINS DIET

Much has been written about this diet and for the overweight person it must sound like **advice from heaven** to try a diet advocating eating almost unlimited meat, eggs, cheese, butter, sausages and bacon whilst discouraging bread, rice and fruit! This diet is basically high in fat and protein but contains very little carbohydrate – no more than 20 grams per day. On the basis of this diet, Atkins published two books entitled "Dr.Atkins Diet Revolution" in 1972 and "Dr.Atkins New Diet Revolution " in 1999, and these together sold about 25 million copies. The reason for this success was undoubtedly because of the huge media hype by the New York Times, CBS and numerous follow-up stories that appeared throughout the USA and eventually in the UK and elsewhere. In addition, many people who tried the Atkins diet reported rapid losses in weight and described him as "a great man". The fat in the Atkins diet was believed to reduce the appetite and stop cravings for carbohydrate.

Figure 1. Showing some of the high fat foods recommended by Atkins

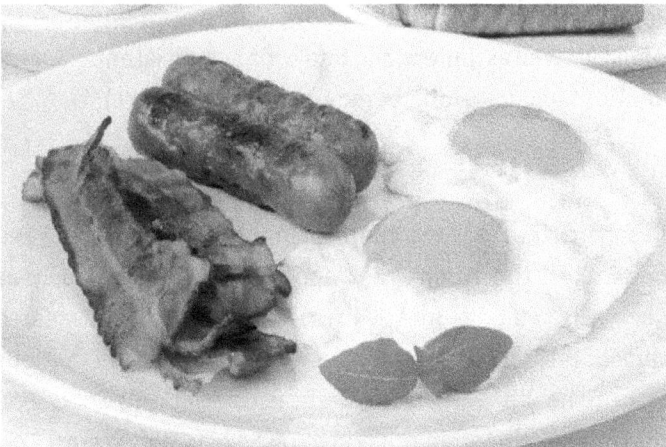

The problem with the Atkins diet is that it is extremely high in animal fats. It also limits the intake of fresh fruit and vegetables and whole grain breads that are the cornerstone of healthy nutrition advocated by the majority of the medical profession. Hence, the "eat five or more servings of fruit and vegetables daily" advised everywhere now.

Common sense should tell us that diets high in animal fat and low in fruit and vegetables would lack essential vitamins and minerals and potentially result in high cholesterol levels in the blood (see, however, "**Final Conclusions on Atkins**", below). Thus, the Atkins diet potentially may increase the risk of cancer, heart disease and osteoporosis (resulting in brittle bones), as well as limiting the intake of beneficial antioxidants from fruit and vegetables (see Chapters 7, 8 of IYL).

These are the reasons that so **many organizations have condemned the Atkins diet** and described it variously as "negligent" and " a massive health risk"(Medical Research Council; British Nutrition Foundation, 2003), and a "serious threat to health" (American Medical Association's Council on Food and Nutrition, submission to US Select Committee,1973) (see reference 14).

BUT IT SEEMS TO WORK for rapid weight loss and this is why so many people have tried it. Unfortunately, the Atkins Diet has been shown to work for a few months but **after one year it has been reported to be less effective than simple low fat diets**. In addition, many people find it difficult to maintain the Atkins diet and drop out. Maybe this is the reason that more people have not been harmed by the extreme nature of the Atkins diet.

FINAL CONCLUSION ON ATKINS. More recently, much has been made of a few studies seemingly supporting the Atkins diet. One example, in 2007, showed that Atkins was effective for weight–loss in 311 women and even after one year had no adverse effects on cholesterol or blood pressure levels (see reference 15). Nobody knows, however, what the potential harmful long-term effects of the Atkins diet are on health. These few studies have to be balanced against the many hundred of reports showing the value of high intakes of fresh fruit, vegetables and whole grains in a balanced diet together with exercise, as described in Chapters 1 and 2 of this book. We all know how conservative the medical profession can be and how people are fed up with contrary advice given by so-called health and diet experts. **The scientific evidence, however, for using the Atkins diet is limited so be safe and follow the advice given in Chapters 1, 2 (above)** and there will be no need for any stressful new fad diets.

GI DIET

Do you really have time to embark on yet another new trendy diet designed to make money for the authors?

The GI diet basically classifies different carbohydrate-containing foods according to their **effect on blood glucose (sugar) levels** once they are digested in the gut. After digestion, glucose is released into the blood from different foods at varying rates. Thus, some foods are rapidly digested and cause **swift rises in blood glucose and have a high GI index**. Other foods are digested slowly and cause only **gradual rises in blood glucose and have a low GI index**.

Foods are often classified as having high, medium or low GI values; glucose itself has a maximum GI of 100. Food charts are available giving the GI values of different foods.

The idea of classifying foods by their GI index is that those with a high GI index will raise blood sugar rapidly so that you will feel tired, lacking in energy and hungry within a short time of eating them. In contrast, those with a low GI index raise blood sugar slowly and provide energy supplies longer so that hunger is delayed and less snacking is likely to occur.

ADVANTAGES OF THE GI DIET are that it has generally had a good reception from health professionals since eating low GI foods helps to prevent rapid fluctuations in blood sugar and may reduce the risk of Type 2 diabetes (non-insulin dependent). In addition, the GI diet may increase levels of "good" cholesterol (HDL cholesterol) in the blood and reduce the incidence of heart problems.

DISADVANTAGES OF THE GI DIET are that some foods do not seem to fit into a healthy lifestyle. Thus, crisps, milk chocolate and salted peanuts are included in the low GI category while Branflakes, Cornflakes and water melon have high GI values. This can all get very confusing. In addition, since different foods are eaten together at a meal, it may be difficult to calculate the GI index of the whole meal. In the real world, most of us do not have the time to calculate or remember GI values or the calorie contents of each meal. What we need is to develop a healthy lifestyle **for the rest of our lives**, realize generally which foods are good or bad, and take plenty of exercise as a norm.

FINAL CONCLUSION ON GI DIETS. Providing that foods with low GI values but high fat levels (salted peanuts, crisps etc) are limited then the GI diet should do no harm and some weight loss can be expected (see reference 16a). Such GI diets will, however, require some considerable menu planning with little advantage over the healthy principles described earlier in this present chapter.

Summary

1. Some fats are good for us while others are bad and associated with heart disease and cancer. Good fats are the **unsaturated mononsaturates and polyunsaturates** found mainly in vegetable oils and margarines made from these, as well as in oily fish like salmon, mackerel, sardines and pilchards (see, Table 1). Bad fats are **the saturated and the trans fatty acids**. Saturated fats are present in full-fat dairy products, fatty meats, sausages,

burgers, pies, biscuits etc. Most trans fats originate in the diet through "processing" by heating vegetable oils together with hydrogen to form trans or "hydrogenated" vegetable oils and are then marketed as margarines and used in biscuits, cakes, fried foods and take-away meals.

2. There are many beneficial effects of sufficient fibre (i.e. 20-25 grams daily) in the diet including reductions in constipation, cancer of the colon, cholesterol levels and heart disease, and it may also help to prevent and control diabetes and weight problems.

3. Avoid fad diets such as Atkins and GI and follow the advice in Chapters 2-3 to control and reduce weight. Since weight control can be problematic joining together with others can reinforce maintenance of a healthy diet and exercise regimen.

The next book in the series is:

It's Your Life – Avoiding Harmful Chemicals in Your Food

For the complete guide to a healthy life:

It's Your Life: End the confusion from inconsistent health advice

Reference sources for conclusions

Chapter 1

1. Giovannucci and colleagues. A prospective study of tomato products, lycopene, and prostate cancer risk. Journal National Cancer Institute, Vol. 94, pages 391–398, 2002.

2. Kavanaugh and colleagues, Journal of the National Cancer Institute, Vol. 99, pages 1074-1085, 2007.

3. Sinha and colleagues, Archives of Internal Medicine, Vol. 169, pages 562-571, 2009.

4. Bochukova, and colleagues. Large, rare chromosomal deletions associated with severe early-onset obesity. Nature 6th December, 2009 (**http://dx.doi.org/10.1038/nature08689**)

5. www.salt.gov.uk/publications.html for a free download of "The Little Book of Salt".

6. Draft Energy Requirements report 'scientific consultation', SACN, November 2009.

Chapter 2

7. www.eatwell.gov.uk/foodlabels/trafficlights

8. www.weightlossresources.co.uk/calories-in-food

9. www.calorieking.com/foods

10. www.tiscali.co.uk/lifestyle/healthfitness/calorie/data

11. Lee and Griffin, Nutrition Bulletin, Vol.31, pages 21-27, 2006.

12. "Fit Not Fat at 40+" (Prevention Health Books, 2004, published by Rodale Inc. (ISBN1-4050-4179-X).

Chapter 3

13. Perspectives in Public Health, Vol. 129, pages 56-57, 2009 (see: http://rsh.sagepub.com)

14. www.atkinsexposed.org for detailed refs on the Atkins Diet.

15. Gardner and colleagues, J. American Medical Association, Vol. 297, pages 969-977, 2007.

16a.Govindji, A. and N. Puddefoot, "The 10-Day Gi Diet", published by Vermillion, UK, 2006.